MINERAL HOMEOSTASIS IN THE ELDERLY

CURRENT TOPICS IN NUTRITION AND DISEASE

Series Editors

Anthony A. Albanese
The Burke Rehabilitation Center
White Plains, New York

David Kritchevsky
The Wistar Institute
Philadelphia, Pennsylvania

MINERAL HOMEOSTASIS IN THE ELDERLY

Proceedings of a Conference to Establish Research Priorities, Held in Durham, North Carolina April 20–21, 1988

Editor

Connie W. Bales
Center for the Study of Aging
and Human Development, and
Division of Geriatric Medicine
Duke University
Durham, North Carolina

Presented by the National Institute on Aging, National Institute of Diabetes, Digestive, and Kidney Diseases, and the Duke University Center for the Study of Aging and Human Development.

Alan R. Liss, Inc., New York

Address all Inquiries to the Publisher
Alan R. Liss, Inc., 41 East 11th Street, New York, NY 10003

Library of Congress Cataloging-in-Publication Data

Mineral homeostasis in the elderly.

(Current topics in nutrition and disease; v. 21)
Based on a conference held on Apr. 20 and 21, 1988,
sponsored jointly by the Duke University Center for
the Study of Aging and Human Development, the National
Institute on Aging, and the National Institute of
Diabetes, Digestive, and Kidney Diseases.
Includes bibliographies and index.
1. Mineral metabolism—Age factors—Congresses.
2. Mineral metabolism—Disorders—Age factors—
Congress. 3. Homeostasis—Congresses. 4. Aged—
Diseases—Congresses. I. Bales, Connie W. II. Duke
University. Center for the Study of Aging and Human
Development. III. National Institute on Aging.
IV. National Institute of Diabetes, Digestive, and
Kidney Diseases (U.S.) V. Series. [DNLM: 1. Calcium—
metabolism—congresses. 2. Homeostasis—in old age—
congresses. 3. Minerals—metabolism—congresses.
WI CU82R v.21 / QU 130 M6653 1988]
QP 533.M55   1988   621'.392   88-8472
ISBN 0-8451-1620-7

Contents

Contributors

H. James Armbrecht, Geriatric Research, Education, and Clinical Center, St. Louis Veterans Administration Medical Center, St. Louis, MO 63125; and Departments of Medicine and Biochemistry, St. Louis University School of Medicine, St. Louis, MO 63104 **[127]**

Connie W. Bales, Center for the Study of Aging and Human Development, and Division of Geriatric Medicine, Duke University Medical Center, Durham, NC 27710 **[ix,3,251]**

Fares F. Behmardi, Graduate Nutrition Division, University of Texas at Austin, Austin, TX 78712 **[141]**

Robert J. Cousins, Center for Nutritional Sciences, University of Florida, Gainesville, FL 32611 **[207]**

Marc K. Drezner, Department of Medicine, Duke University Medical Center, Durham, NC 27710 **[245,251]**

Deborah T. Gold, Center for the Study of Aging and Human Development, and Department of Psychiatry, Duke University Medical Center, Durham, NC 27710 **[251]**

Jeanne H. Freeland-Graves, Division of Graduate Nutrition, University of Texas at Austin, Austin, TX 78712 **[3,107,141]**

Janet L. Greger, Department of Nutritional Sciences, University of Wisconsin, Madison, WI 53706 **[171]**

Robert P. Heaney, Creighton University, Omaha, NE 68178 **[115]**

Pao-Hwa Lin, Division of Graduate Nutrition, University of Texas at Austin, Austin, TX 78712 **[107]**

Kenneth W. Lyles, Department of Medicine, Duke University Medical Center, and Geriatric Research, Education, and Clinical Center, Veterans Administration Medical Center, Durham, NC 27710 **[251]**

Ananda S. Prasad, Department of Medicine, Division of Hematology-Oncology, Wayne State University School of Medicine, Harper–Grace Hospitals, Detroit, MI 48201; and United States Veterans Administration Medical Center, Allen Park, MI 48101 **[69,201]**

The numbers in brackets are the opening page numbers of the contributors' articles.

P. Isaac Rabbani, Department of Medicine, Wayne State University School of Medicine, and United States Veterans Administration Medical Center, Allen Park, MI 48101; present address: Department of Toxicology, Food and Drug Administration, Washington, DC 20204 **[201]**

Noel W. Solomons, Center for Studies of Sensory Impairment, Aging and Metabolism, National Committee for the Blind and Deaf of Guatemala, Hospital de Ojos Y Oidos "Dr. Rodolfo Robles V", Zona 11, Guatemala City, Guatemala **[35]**

William P. Steffee, Saint Vincent Charity Hospital, Cleveland, OH 44115 **[223]**

J. Carlos Teran, Saint Vincent Charity Hospital, Cleveland, OH 44115 **[223]**

Robert H. Wasserman, Department of Physiology, Cornell University, New York State College of Veterinary Medicine, Ithaca, NY 14853 **[15]**

Preface

Improvements in public health and medical care have greatly extended the longevity of Americans during this century. With average life expectancy at an all time high, the quality of life, rather than its length, has become the issue of foremost importance to many persons of middle age and older. More and more, we witness the search for ways to maintain good health and "add life to our years."

Many factors that influence health status are determined before birth. Sex, body type, and genetic predisposition to specific disease states cannot be altered. In contrast, nutritional status is a highly malleable parameter of health and well-being. Thus we find that nutritional modification of health and longevity is a topic that has recently enjoyed a surge of interest in both the scientific community and among lay people. Despite this increased attention, surprisingly little is known about the specific nutritional needs of the elderly, especially regarding metabolism and requirements for micronutrients.

Because of this paucity of information, nutrition scientists face a critical need to extend the boundaries of knowledge concerning the interaction of nutrition with the aging process. This can only be done by formulating sound research hypotheses regarding nutrition and aging and testing them in well-designed and carefully executed experimental and clinical studies. The essential first step in this process is the definition of research priorities for immediate and long–term study.

The purpose of this book is to focus attention on age-related alterations in the metabolism of essential mineral nutrients. This publication is the result of a conference jointly sponsored by the Duke University Center for the Study of Aging and Human Development, the National Institute on Aging, and the National Institute of Diabetes, Digestive, and Kidney Diseases. A major objective of the conference was to define current understanding of mineral homeostasis in the elderly and to establish research priorities for future studies in this field.

For certain minerals such as calcium and iron, which have already been the subject of considerable research, it is clear that future studies should focus on the specifics of age-related changes in requirements and metabolism. The discussions of bone architecture and of innovative approaches to the treatment of osteoporosis in this text are examples of efforts to move beyond current understanding and to address the complexities of age-related changes in mineral metabolism. In the case of trace minerals, for which there is a striking shortage of data concerning adults of all ages, we face the formidable task of defining the specifics of mineral homeostasis in maturity before we can explore alterations that may occur as individuals age. Thus the chapters that concern trace mineral metabolism consider the current state of the art as well as needs for future studies of age-associated alterations in mineral homeostasis. The potential interaction of age-related chronic disease (and requisite therapy) with mineral status is an underlying theme in a number of these chapters.

This volume is organized into three parts. The first addresses specific mechanisms which maintain mineral homeostasis; it focuses on dietary requirements, intestinal uptake, and metabolism of minerals in the elderly. The second part concerns alterations in mineral metabolism that occur as a consequence of aging. Papers in the third part address the interaction of chronic illness with mineral status and the potential for nutritional intervention in disorders of mineral homeostasis. To emphasize the importance of research, a related "research summary" follows each of the three parts; these brief reports are based on research presented at the Duke University conference.

Mineral homeostasis clearly interacts with age and with many chronic diseases that occur with increased prevalence in older adults. It is the hope of the contributors that conferences such as the one which preceded this publication will encourage the exchange of information and ideas and promote a rapid but carefully focused increase in research studies concerning mineral homeostasis in the elderly.

During the time that this book was being prepared for publication, the field of nutrition suffered the loss of two preeminent scientists, Dr. Lucille Hurley and Dr. Henry Kamin. Both were greatly interested in many of the topics addressed in this book. Its publication serves as a tribute to their unique contributions to the study of nutrition.

In addition to the previously mentioned sponsors, we would like to acknowledge the assistance provided by the administrative staff of the Duke University Center for the Study of Aging and Human Development and the production staff at Alan R. Liss, Inc., for their dedicated efforts toward the timely production of this text.

Connie W. Bales

NORMAL MINERAL HOMEOSTASIS AND AGING

Mineral Homeostasis in the Elderly, pages 3–14
© *1989 Alan R. Liss, Inc.*

DIETARY RECOMMENDATIONS OF MINERALS FOR THE ELDERLY

Jeanne H. Freeland-Graves and Connie W. Bales

Graduate Nutrition Division, University of Texas at Austin, Austin, Texas 78712 and Center for the Study of Aging, Duke University Medical Center, Durham, North Carolina 27710

The recommended dietary allowances (RDAs) serve as guidelines for daily intakes of nutrients that healthy population groups in the United States should have in their diets. The levels specified are generous since they are designed for groups, not individuals. Since the RDAs have been established to meet the needs of 97.5% of the population, individuals who ingest levels less than the RDA may not necessarily be at risk for a given nutrient. However, it is believed that continual intakes below the RDA increase the likelihood that the diet is nutritionally inadequate.

In the United States, the Food and Nutrition Board of the National Research Council (1980) has established RDAs for three macrominerals (calcium, magnesium, and phosphorus) and three trace elements (zinc, iron, and iodine). For other minerals that are known to be dietary essentials for humans, a lack of quantitative data has prevented the creation of specific RDAs. Instead, a separate category called estimated safe and adequate daily dietary intakes (ESADDIs) has been established. The ESADDIs have upper as well as lower limits since certain trace elements can be toxic. Trace minerals for which an ESADDI has been set include copper, manganese, fluoride, chromium, selenium, and molybdenum. A number of other trace elements may also be essential for humans, such as cobalt, nickel, vanadium, silicon, tin, arsenic, cadmium, and boron. However, with few exceptions (Johnson and Greger, 1982; Nielsen et al., 1987; Carlisle, 1978), research on human requirements for these nutrients to date is virtually nonexistent.

This chapter summarizes the current understanding of recommended intakes of minerals for the elderly and emphasizes the need for further study of their requirements in this age group. Specific minerals are discussed only briefly in this paper. The reader is referred to subsequent chapters in this text for detailed examinations of absorption, metabolism, requirement, and deficiency of essential minerals in the elderly.

DIETARY RECOMMENDATIONS IN AGING

It is well known that the amount of lean body mass declines with age and that this change is accompanied by a concomitant increase in adipose tissue (Food and Nutrition Board, 1980). Since adipose tissue has a lower metabolic rate than lean body mass, this extra proportion of body fat to protein diminishes energy requirements as one ages. The decrease in basal metabolic rate is estimated to be approximately 2% per decade after the age of 21. In addition, levels of physical activity almost always diminish with aging. The result is an age-associated reduction in caloric needs.

If an individual fails to reduce caloric intakes with advancing age, weight gain is the normal consequence. This decline in energy requirements with aging has led the Food and Nutrition Board to establish four categories of energy requirements for adults: 19-22, 23-50, 51-75 and 76+ years.

But do requirements for other nutrients, such as minerals, also change with aging? We do not know the answer to this question. In 1980, the Food and Nutrition Board divided the RDAs for adults into three age groups: 19-22, 23-50, and 51+ years. It is proposed that the next revision of the RDAs will have adult categories which will include the elderly. Older individuals will be divided into 51-75 and 76+ yrs. The ESADDIs for other nutrients have only one category for all adults.

With the exception of a reduction in iron for postmenopausal women, no adjustments have been made for recommendations concerning mineral intakes with aging even though metabolism and/or body pool size may vary. Studies upon which current adult recommendations are based have used primarily young or middle-aged subjects, with extrapolation of results to older age groups. The justification for this extrapolation is lacking, since nutritional needs of the elderly may reflect decades of previous nutrient intake, as well as the impact of physiological changes generally unique to old age. Moreover, the dramatic heterogeneity of older adults makes it difficult to derive dietary recommendations even for "normal" elderly.

For certain minerals, there is substantial evidence that body needs may be greater with advancing age. The current RDA for calcium, for example, is 800 mg per day for all adults. Yet persuasive studies (Heaney et al., 1978) have led experts in the field to recommend higher calcium intakes for both peri- and post-menopausal women (Consensus Conference Statement on Osteoporosis, 1984). Special recommendations for those with osteoporosis, a bone disease which affects 25-35 million older Americans, may also be necessary (Avioli, 1987).

Another mineral that may also be particularly important for elderly individuals is zinc. The role of zinc in the immune function of the human

(Duchateau et al., 1981; Bogden et al., 1987) suggests that this nutrient is critical for the elderly, who often have a multitude of illnesses.

Very little is known about the specific needs of the elderly for the ultratrace elements, such as silicon, boron, chromium, and manganese. However, ample preliminary evidence exists for potentially important roles for many of these nutrients in the health of older adults (Carlisle, 1978; Nielsen et al., 1987; Mertz, 1986; Strause and Saltman, 1987).

There is a clear need to quantify recommendations for various age groups, but this problem has not been resolved due to a lack of available information. Several other countries have recognized this dilemma and established a greater number of age categories (Truswell, 1983). Japan, for example, has eight categories of dietary recommendations for adults, including one for age 19-20, and then one for each decade of life up to the age of 80+ years. Three countries (Bulgaria, Singapore, Thailand) have six categories of dietary recommendations for adults while nine countries (Bolivia, Caribbean, Columbia, Italy, Malaysia, Phillipines, Spain, Uruguay, Venezuela) have five categories. Presumably the United States has limited the number of categories for advanced age because of the paucity of data.

BASIS FOR SETTING DIETARY RECOMMENDATIONS

Dietary recommendations are generally derived from individual nutrient requirements. A nutrient requirement is defined as the amount necessary to meet the physiological needs of an individual such that one remains in good health. However, extrapolation of a nutrient requirement of an individual to a population is difficult because of variability in individual biochemistry, anthropometrics, and social, economic, and geographic environment as well as incidence of infection and chronic disease.

It is also difficult to apply the theoretical requirements obtained under strict laboratory conditions to the daily environment. We must remember that people eat foods in the form of meals and rarely ingest single nutrients. Factors in foods such as phytates, fiber, oxalates and the presence of other nutrients may significantly alter the absorption, retention, metabolism and/or excretion of a mineral, and hence, the dietary requirement. Furthermore, it is believed that humans may be able to adapt to relatively low levels of micronutrient intake. For example, Africans and Asians have been reported to maintain healthy bones on calcium intakes of 500 mg/day while Europeans are usually in negative balance on intakes of 800 mg/day (Truswell,1983).

However, the ability to adapt to a wide range of nutrient intakes may be age-dependent. The "homeostenosis" of old age suggested by Rowe (1986) may reduce the adaptive capacity of the elderly and thus jeopardize nutritional homeostasis when intakes are marginally deficient or excessive. For example, excretion may be increased for those minerals that are excreted primarily by the kidney since renal function may decline with aging (Solomons, 1986). Whether or not age-related decrements in kidney function could reduce the ability to maintain homeostasis even with seemingly adequate levels of nutrients is unclear.

METHODS OF ASSESSING DIETARY REQUIREMENTS

Currently, there is no one method that is able to determine nutrient requirements precisely. Methods used for assessment of human requirements include: (1) levels of dietary intakes related to the health of a population or (2) the appearance of a deficiency disease; (3) long-term balance studies that determine the minimal amount needed to maintain positive balance in both healthy individuals and patients on total parenteral nutrition; (4) isotope kinetics; (5) absorption studies; and (6) supplementation studies of the amount needed to alleviate clinical signs of a deficiency; (7) saturate tissues; or (8) to provide normal function for an assessment parameter. Parameters of assessment may include serum or plasma levels of the nutrient itself and/or related enzymes and, more recently, functional indicators such as the immune response.

Relating Dietary Intakes to Health

The initial step taken by most nutritionists to determine requirements is to observe levels of dietary nutrients that maintain the health of a population. Baseline data must be gathered on levels in typical diets and related to records of morbidity and moribundity. Yet for several trace elements, it is impossible to obtain these data since tables of food composition are either incomplete or nonexistent. A real need exists for developing more complete composition tables of trace elements in foods.

But it should be emphasized that total dietary intakes that meet the RDAs are not always assurances of nutritional adequacy. Consideration must be given to differences in the form of the mineral, such as heme vs. nonheme iron (Nordstrom, 1982) and the amount and type of dietary components that affect bioavailability. These dietary components include ascorbic acid (Monsen and Cook, 1976), tannins (polyphenols), phytates (Bales et al., 1987), and fiber, as well as interacting nutrients such as manganese vs. calcium (Lin and Freeland-Graves, this volume) or iron (Freeland-Graves et al., 1986).

The adequacy of nutrient intakes is also dependent on the nutritional and health status of the subjects studied. Absorption of iron, for example, is believed to be an inverse function of iron status and thus, absorption increases substantially as body stores decline (Lynch et al., 1982). In individuals with chronic infections and diseases, the absorption, metabolism, and excretion of trace elements can be dramatically altered.

It is estimated that 85% of all Americans over age 65 have at least one chronic disease (National Center for Health Statistics, 1982). These elderly often take multiple over-the-counter and prescription drugs. A number of these drugs are known to bind to trace elements and render them biologically unavailable or exhibit other adverse effects. For example, extensive use of aspirin can lead to intestinal bleeding and concomitant losses of nutrients in blood. It is possible that the recent publicity over the preventative role of aspirin in heart attacks may lead to excessive use by some elderly to the point that iron needs are affected. The extent to which drug use in the elderly affects mineral requirements is an area that is totally unexplored.

One other factor that could influence the utilization of otherwise adequate dietary intakes is a reduction in gastric acidity. This reduction in acidity is a problem for a number of elderly who have age-related atrophic gastritis or partial or complete gastrectomies. Also, antacid use is common in this age group and such a practice can diminish the acidity of the gastrointestinal tract (Schlenker, 1984). Bioavailability of minerals could be lowered in such a condition since an acidic pH is required for optimal absorption of several minerals, e.g. calcium and iron (Russell, 1986).

In summary, the presence of any of the above factors makes it impossible to assess nutritional status and requirements from diet alone. Furthermore, after quantities of nutrient intakes have been established, these must be related to the nutrient and health status of a population. Yet in many cases, diagnostic indicators of nutritional status are not available nor have they been verified for accuracy. It is imperative that additional parameters of mineral status be developed in order to accurately assess potential nutritional problems.

Balance Studies

Since optimal nutrient status is the result of achieving a positive balance between the intake and excretion of a nutrient, balance studies are one way of determining if a particular level of dietary intake is sufficient to maintain positive balance. However, there are many problems associated with this technique.

Perhaps the most common mistake made by researchers is a failure to conduct these types of studies on a long-term basis. Short-term balance studies have little validity since fecal mixing of dietary constituents may occur for 1-2 weeks after the start of a study. In order to separate out the effect of the previous diet or treatment, the excreta for the initial time period must be discarded. Unfortunately, some investigators still conduct one week balance studies, making it impossible to adequately assess the influence of the treatment studied and the implications of the results.

An error associated with balance studies that is often overlooked is the wide variability in the body status of the mineral to be studied. Individual differences in mineral status may greatly influence responses to the dietary levels fed to balance study participants (Freeland-Graves et al., 1988). Although the human has a remarkable ability to adapt to varying nutrient intakes, it is difficult to quantify the effect of adaptation on mineral balance. As previously noted, iron is regulated primarily by absorption, which is, in turn, regulated by body stores of the mineral (Lynch et al., 1982). Thus, subjects who differ in iron status will produce variable responses to a given dietary intake of the mineral. The heterogeneity of humans and their diets is a confounding factor that is inherent in all human studies.

Another problem in using balance data for determining mineral requirements is that the amount of the mineral retained in the body may increase as the dietary level increases (Freeland-Graves et al., 1987). For some minerals, such as manganese (Friedman et al., 1987), endogenous losses through bile, pancreatic and intestinal secretions may vary considerably depending on the need and ability of the body to conserve or eliminate the nutrient. Thus, studies which feed high dietary levels of a mineral may result in much higher requirements than that needed on a lower mineral intake. The opposite may also be true.

One balance method that has been used to estimate endogenous losses is the feeding of a depletion diet, followed by repletion (Friedman et al., 1987; Hess et al., 1977; Levander et al., 1981). Measurements of fecal, urinary and integumental losses when the amount in the diet is negligible will provide some indication of the amount of the mineral that is excreted and, presumably, must be replaced. However, obligatory losses of minerals may be lower than normal with this technique because of a need to conserve body stores during a deficiency. Or endogenous losses could be higher than normal since depletion diets are typically semi-purified and do not contain the usual inhibitory factors that bind trace elements as found in conventional foods. Binding of bile to the variety of fibers and phytates found in typical diets would reduce the amount of enterohepatic circulation and could lead to high endogenous losses via bile.Thus, data derived from studies using deficiency levels of a nutrient may not be definitive for estimating daily requirements.

Newer methods of estimating requirements include balance studies of patients receiving total parenteral nutrition (TPN) (Shike et al., 1981; Anderson et al., 1988). This method may be ideal for determining endogenous losses for some minerals, such as zinc and iron, since administering excess of the nutrient intravenously has been reported not to increase the amount excreted (Jeejeebhoy, 1986). Whether or not this is true for the other minerals is unknown but deserves further investigation.

One disadvantage in using TPN patients for estimating requirements is that they may have suboptimal health or have abnormal body functions and/or structure. However, collections of endogenous mineral losses from these patients can provide valuable information and this type of study should be utilized more frequently in the future.

Isotope kinetics

Another valid method of estimating requirements is by studying the kinetics of radioisotope uptake and distribution in tissues, such as blood (Green et al., 1968). However, uniform labeling of the body mineral is imperative before measurements of the isotope are valid and this may take several years (Lynch et al., 1982). Also, care must be taken that the individuals studied are representative of the population since the sample size will be small.

Dual isotopes are often used to quantify the contribution of endogenous losses to total fecal output. In this method, one isotope is administered intravenously while the other is given orally. Any of the intravenously administered isotope that is found in the excreta is assumed to be derived from endogenous losses. For ethical reasons, stable isotopes are often the ideal way to measure endogenous losses but these may be cost prohibitive or unavailable. For example, this technique is impossible for manganese since the trace mineral is monoisotopic.

Absorption studies

Once estimates of endogenous losses have been quantified, this information must be combined with accurate absorption values in order to provide a recommended dietary level. Yet data on intestinal absorption of nutrients is subject to inaccuracy since that derived from giving pulse doses of a miniscule quantity of an element in fasting subjects may not accurately reflect the real life situation in which individuals consume larger amounts in diets full of inhibitory and/or accelerating factors (phytates, fiber, ascorbic acid, other minerals). The ideal way to measure absorption of trace minerals is via stable isotopes incorporated into diets fed for a period of time. Yet only a limited number of studies (Turnland et al., 1982a ; 1982b) have used this technique in the elderly.

In aging, absorption of minerals may decrease as a result of morphological changes in the brush border membrane, diminished secretion of digestive enzymes, or metabolic alterations in nutrient transport mechanisms. One example of the latter would be the reduction in calcium uptake that would occur with a decline in the activation of vitamin D due to dysfunction of the liver and/or kidney. Whether these alterations are great enough to significantly affect balance and, ultimately, body stores is unknown.

Response to Supplementation of a Nutrient

The most definitive approach for documenting possible mineral deficiencies in a population would be to assess the response to an oral supplement (Lynch et al., 1982). Responses could include the amount needed to alleviate clinical symptoms of a deficiency, saturate body tissues or fluids, or to provide normal function of established assessment parameters. This method would enable one to establish levels of dietary intakes that appear to be sufficient for nutritional adequacy. However, the first approach cannot be undertaken with subclinical deficiencies since the deficiency must be advanced enough to be expressed via a clinical symptom. The second approach is time-consuming and it is unclear whether saturation of body tissues is always a desirable condition. Finally, the third approach may be limited for many trace minerals until more precise indicators of body status are developed.

TYPES OF DIETARY RECOMMENDATIONS

The use of a range of levels (as in the ESADDIs) rather than only one figure (as in the RDAs) may actually be a better way of expressing dietary recommendations. Setting up only one value as the standard for a nutrient invariably leads to disagreement among nutritionists. Do we need to provide: (a) a minimal level needed for prevention of deficiency diseases; (b) an acceptable level for planning most normal diets; (c) the desirable level that would maintain *optimal* rather than simply adequate health; and/or (d) a toxic level as well?

The creation of separate recommendations for each of these four conditions might alleviate confusion. A *minimum* level could be used by health personnel and nutritionists for assessment of the degree of nutritional adequacy of diets. An *acceptable* level could be used by dietitians for planning nutritionally adequate meals for groups, governments for evaluating national food supplies, and industry for nutrition labelling.

A *desirable* level could be used by consumers who want to minimize the risk of degenerative diseases such as cancer, cardiovascular disease, and stroke. Although it can be argued that disease prevention is not a concern for "normal adults", it is clear that consumers are interested in the latest information concerning the role of nutrition in optimal health and disease prevention. This information could be reflected in the "desirable" intake levels and be updated as new results are available.

Finally, a *toxic* level could be used by consumers and manufacturers as guidelines for limiting daily intakes of nutrients. The establishment of a toxic level for certain elements is critical, since it may be relatively easy to overdose with amounts that are only several-fold greater than usual dietary intakes.

The idea that a different set of standards be formulated for varying purposes is not new. In 1975, Hegsted (1975) declared that one set of standards could not be used to evaluate both food consumption records and the planning of diets and food supplies. In 1983, Truswell suggested three categories be used for dietary standards: a *low diagnostic level* to be used by health professionals to assess nutrient adequacy; a *recommended dietary intake* to be used by dietitians and consumers for meal planning; and an *upper level* to indicate possible adverse effects.

Only a limited number of countries have implemented multiple standards for dietary recommendations. For example, Australia has adopted the use of the three above standards, but has used a range of intakes, rather than just one value, for the recommended dietary intakes (Palmer, 1982). Two other countries have established additional standards. New Zealand has both a *minimum safe intake* as well as an *adequate daily intake*. Scandinavia has an additional *low diagnostic level*. The establishment of a set of standards for each mineral is an idea that should be given further consideration. The specific terminology used for each level is probably less important than the recognition that a single value or RDA cannot adequately express all the factors now known to be relevant to the intake of a given nutrient.

CONCLUSIONS

With the exception of iron, adjustments of dietary recommendations for aging have not been made for minerals since there is a lack of adequate data available. Whether diminished lean body mass and/or other age-related metabolic changes are of sufficient magnitude to suggest changes in dietary intakes for the elderly is generally unknown. Dietary recommendations are developed from nutrient requirements. However, no one method of determining mineral requirements is problem-free. Thus, a variety of methods must be utilized and the results compiled to produce a consensus. It is suggested that researchers seek to establish four sets of dietary recommendations: the minimum, acceptable, desirable and toxic levels. Once these recommendations have been established, modifications for the impact of aging must be incorporated. However, it is clear that further research concerning mineral requirements of the elderly must precede the development of these age-specific recommendations.

ACKNOWLEDGMENTS:

This work was supported in part by U. S. Department of Agriculture Competitive Research Grant 87-CRCR-1-2312 and University Research Institute, Biomedical Research Support Grant RR07-091-21 to the first author; and National Institute on Aging Grants AG00029 and AGO7494 to the second author.

REFERENCES

Anderson RA, Borel JS, Polansky MM, Bryden NA, Majerus TC, Moser PB (1988). Chromium intake and excretion of patients receiving total parenteral nutrition. Effects of supplemental chromium. J Trace Elem Exper Med 1: 9-18.
Avioli LV (1987). The calcium controversy and the Recommended Dietary Allowance. In Avioli L V (ed) : "The Osteoporotic Syndrome: Detection, Prevention, and Treatment," Orlando, FL: Grune & Stratton, Inc., pp 57-66.
Bales CW, Freeland-Graves JH, Lin P-H, Stone J, Dougherty V (1987). Plasma uptake of manganese: response to dose and dietary factors. In Kies C (ed) : "Nutritional Bioavailability of Manganese," Washington, DC: American Chemical Society, pp 112-122.
Bogden JD, Oleske JM, Munves EM, Lavenhar MA, Bruening KS, Kemp FW, Holding KJ, Denny TN, Louria DB (1987). Zinc and immunocompetence in the elderly: Baseline data on zinc nutriture and immunity in unsupplemented subjects. Am J Clin Nutr 46: 101-109.
Carlisle E (1978). In Bendz G and Lindqvist I (eds) : "Biochemistry of Silicon and Related Problems", New York: Plenum Press, pp 231-252.
Consensus Conference Statement on Osteoporosis (1984). J Am Med Assoc 252: 799-802.

Duchateau J, Delepesse G, Vrijens R, Collet H (1981). Beneficial effects of oral zinc supplementation on the immune response of old people. Am J Med 70: 1001-1004.

Food and Nutrition Board (1980). Recommended Dietary Allowances, 9th Ed. Washington, DC: National Academy of Sciences.

Freeland-Graves JH, Bales CW, Behmardi FB (1987). Manganese requirements in humans. In Kies C (ed) : "Nutritional Bioavailability of Manganese," Washington, DC: American Chemical Society, pp 90-104.

Freeland-Graves JH, Behmardi F, Bales CW, Dougherty V, Lin P-H, Crosby JB, Trickett PC (1988). Metabolic balance in young men consuming diets containing five levels of dietary manganese. J Nutr 118: 764-773.

Freeland-Graves JH, Lin P-H, Dougherty V, Bales CW (1986). The influence of iron and ascorbic acid on the plasma uptake of manganese. First Meeting of the International Society for Trace Element Research in Humans, p 56.

Friedman BJ, Freeland-Graves JH, Bales CW, Behmardi FB, Shorey-Kutschke R, Willis RA, Crosby JB, Trickett PC, Houston SD (1987). Manganese balance and clinical observations in young men fed a manganese deficient diet. J Nutr 117: 133-143.

Green R, Charlton RW, Seftel H, Bothwell TH, Mayet F, Adams EB, Finch CA, Layrisse M (1968). Body iron excretion in man. A collaborative study. Am J Med 45: 336-353.

Heaney RP, Recker RR, Saville PD (1978). Menopausal changes in calcium balance performance. J Lab Clin Med 92: 953-963.

Hegsted DM (1975). Dietary standards. J Am Dietet Assoc 66: 13-21.

Hess FM, King JC, Margen S (1977). Zinc excretion in young women fed low zinc intakes and oral contraceptives. J Nutr 107: 1610-1620.

Jeejeebhoy KN (1986). Nutritional balance studies: indicators of human requirement or adaptive mechanisms. J Nutr 116: 2061-2063.

Johnson MA, Greger JL (1982). Effects of dietary tin and calcium metabolism of adult males. Am J Clin Nutr 35: 655-660.

Levander OA, Sutherland B, Morris VC, King JC (1981). Selenium balance in young men during selenium depletion and repletion. Am J Clin Nutr 34: 2662-2669.

Lin P-H, Freeland-Graves JH (1988). Effects of simultaneous ingestion of calcium and manganese in humans. In Bales C (ed) : "Mineral Homeostasis in the Elderly," New York: Alan R. Liss.

Lynch SR, Finch CA, Monsen ER, Cook JD (1982). Iron status of elderly Americans. Am J Clin Nutr 36: 1032-1045.

Mertz W (1986). Trace elements and the needs of the elderly. In Hutchinson ML, Munro HN (eds) : "Nutrition and Aging," Orlando, FL: Academic Press, Inc., pp 71-83.

Monsen ER, Cook JD (1976). Food iron absorption in human subjects IV. The effects of calcium and phosphate salts on the absorption of nonheme iron. Am J Clin Nutr 29: 1142-1148.

National Center for Health Statistics (1982). "Statistics - Health, United States, 1982. DHHS Pub. No. (PHS) 83-1232," Washington, DC: U.S. Department of Health and Human Services, December.

Nielsen FH, Hunt CD, Mullen LM, Hunt JR (1987). Effect of dietary boron on mineral, estrogen, and testosterone metabolism in postmenopausal women. Proc Soc Exp Biol Med 1: 394-397.

Nordstrom JW (1982). Trace mineral nutrition in the elderly. Am J Clin Nutr 36: 788-795.

Palmer N (1982). Recommended dietary intakes for use in Australia. J Food Nutr 39: 157-193.

Rowe JW (1986). Physiologic interface of aging and nutrition. In Hutchinson M L and Munro H N (eds) : "Nutrition and Aging," Orlando, FL: Academic Press, Inc., pp 11-21.

Russell RM (1986). Implications of gastric atrophy for vitamin and mineral nutriture. In Hutchinson M L and Munro H N (eds.): "Nutrition and Aging," Orlando, FL: Academic Press, Inc., pp 59-69.

Schlenker, E (1984). Nutrition in Aging. St. Louis, Missouri: Times Mirror/Mosby p. 116.

Strause L, Saltman P (1987). Role of manganese in bone metabolism. In Kies C (ed) : "Nutritional Bioavailability of Manganese," Washington, DC: American Chemical Society, pp 46-55.

Shike M, Roulet M, Kurian R, Whitwell J, Stewart S, Jeejeebhoy KN (1981). Copper metabolism and requirements in total parenteral nutrition. Gastroenter 81: 290-297.

Solomons N (1986). Trace elements in nutrition of the elderly 1. Established RDAs for iron, zinc, and iodine. Postgrad Med 79: 231-242.

Truswell AS (1983). Recommended dietary intakes around the world - Introduction. Nutr Abs Rev Clin Nutr - Series A 53: 940-1015.

Turnlund JR, Michel MC, Keyes WR, King JC, Margen S (1982a). Use of enriched stable isotopes to determine zinc and iron absorption in elderly men. Am J Clin Nutr 35: 1033-1040.

Turnlund JR, Michel MC, Keyes WR, Schutz Y, Margen S (1982b). Copper absorption in elderly men determined by using stable ^{65}Cu. Am J Clin Nutr 36: 587-591.

Mineral Homeostasis in the Elderly, pages 15–34

PHYSIOLOGICAL MECHANISMS OF CALCIUM ABSORPTION AND HOMEOSTASIS, WITH EMPHASIS ON VITAMIN D ACTION

Robert H. Wasserman
Cornell University
Dept./Sect. of Physiology
New York State College of Veterinary Medicine
Ithaca, NY 14853

Calcium is required for the optimal and proper functioning of all tissues and organs in humans and other animals, and its multifunctional roles are becoming increasingly appreciated from on-going biomedical research. The skeleton, containing 99% of the body's calcium, owes its hardness and homeostatic function to the presence of calcium phosphate salts within its organic matrix. Calcium is also essential for nerve impulse transmission, muscle contraction, blood coagulation, the secretion of hormones and neurotransmitters, cell growth, motility, replication, as an activator of a number of enzymes, and for cell membrane integrity.

In order to assure that sufficient calcium is available for cell functioning, homeostatic regulators have evolved to maintain blood calcium at a nearly constant concentration of about 2.5 mM (total). The primary regulators of calcium homeostasis are the calcium-regulating hormones; parathyroid hormone, calcitonin, and the hormonal form of vitamin D, 1,25-dihydroxyvitamin D. These hormones act singly or in concert on intestinal Ca^{2+} absorption, bone Ca^{2+} resorption and renal Ca^{2+} reabsorption to achieve plasma calcium homeostasis. Fig. 1 places emphasis on the homeostatic function of the vitamin D hormone.

The free intracellular Ca^{2+} concentration of resting cells is closely controlled at about $10^{-7}M$, a concentration about 10,000 fold lower than the extracellular fluid calcium concentration (Rega, 1985). The resting free calcium concentration is achieved through the coordinate action of several components of the cell (Fig. 1). Calcium can enter the cell by diffusion across the plasma membrane, through potential-activated channels, or through

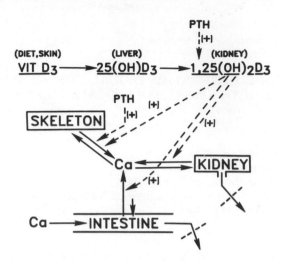

Fig. 1. Vitamin D and Calcium Homeostasis. Vitamin D_3, from dietary sources or from ultraviolet light catalyzed synthesis in the skin, is converted in the liver to the $25(OH)D_3$ and in the kidney to $1,25(OH)_2D_3$. The $1,25(OH)_2D_3$ metabolite participates in the maintenance of serum Ca^{2+} levels by increasing Ca^{2+} absorption from the intestine, increasing the reabsorption of Ca^{2+} from renal tubules and increasing removal of calcium from bone in concert with the parathyroid hormone (PTH). Parathyroid hormone, in addition its bone resorptive function, stimulates the synthesis of $1,25(OH)_2D_3$. The secretion of parathyroid hormone is elevated during periods of hypocalcemia and depressed during periods of normocalcemia and hypercalcemia. The serum Ca^{2+}-parathyroid hormone-$1,25(OH)_2D_3$ axis represents a major component of calcium homeostasis and the feed-back regulation of serum Ca^{2+} concentrations. (Not shown is the PTH effect on increasing urinary phosphate excretion.)

receptor-operated channels. Extrusion of calcium from the cell is the function of an ATP-dependent active Ca^{2+} transport system, and also occurs by sodium-calcium exchange. Further control of the intracellular Ca^{2+} concentration is due to sequestration by the endoplasmic or sarcoplasmic reticulum, the Golgi apparatus, mitochondria and by binding to high affinity calcium-binding macromolecules.

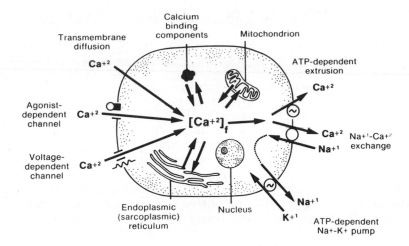

Fig. 2. <u>The Control of Intracellular Calcium.</u> Depicted are cellular components participating in the control of free intracellular $[Ca^{+2}]_f$ at concentrations of about $10^{-7}M$. Calcium enters cells by diffusion across the plasma membrane, and through potential-activated and receptor-activated channels. Extrusion of Ca^{2+} from cells occurs by an ATP-dependent uphill transporting pump and by Na^+/Ca^{2+} exchange. Intracellular Ca^{2+} is further controlled by sequestration and release from the endoplasmic or sarcoplasmic reticulum, mitochondria, other intracellular organelles and various Ca^{2+} binding components.

The role of calcium as a second messenger in the control of cell metabolism has received considerable attention recently (Berridge and Irvine, 1984; Nishizuka, 1986; Rasmussen, 1986; Williamson et al., 1985). Various agonists were shown to activate a specific phospholipase C which initiates a cascade of reactions from the hydrolysis of phosphoinositides. Formed therefrom is inositol-1,4,5-trisphosphate (IP3), a substance that causes the release of Ca^{2+} from an intracellular compartment, considered to be the endoplasmic reticulum. The Ca^{2+} released from the cytosolic compartment transiently increases the concentration of ionic Ca^{2+} within the cell which, through calcium-receptor proteins such as calmodulin, can stimulate the activity of a number of Ca^{2+}-dependent enzymes (e.g., adenylate cyclase, phosphodiesterase, kinases, phosphorylase). The other product of phosphoinositide hydrolysis is diacylglycerol, an activator of protein kinase C, a Ca^{2+}-dependent enzyme.

INTESTINAL ABSORPTION OF CALCIUM: GENERAL FEATURES

Dietary calcium is the only source of this essential cation for land-based animals. To assure that adequate absorption of ingested calcium takes place, specific transport processes are present in the enterocyte. These include uphill, energy dependent calcium transport first disclosed from the in vitro studies of Schachter and Rosen (1959) and Harrison and Harrison (1960), and verified by the use of biophysical in situ procedures with rat (Wasserman et al., 1961) and chick (Wasserman and Kallfelz, 1962) intestine. In addition to the active transport process, calcium is absorbed by a diffusion-like process (Wasserman and Taylor, 1969) in which the rate of calcium absorption is directly related to the intraluminal concentration of calcium. The active transport process saturates at an intracellular calcium concentration of about 2-5 mM (loc cit).

The absorption of calcium occurs in all segments of the small intestine although the efficiency of absorption follows the order: of duodenum > jejunum > ileum (Pansu et al., 1983). Calcium absorption also takes place in the colon (Grinstead et al., 1984; Favus and Langman, 1984; Amman et al., 1986) and cecum (Favus and Backman, 1985).

The two component system of calcium absorption, i.e., a saturable component and a non-saturable component, was evident from the detailed studies of Pansu et al.,(1981) and Toverud and Dostal (1986). The assumption is made, with supporting evidence, that the non-saturable component represents transfer of Ca^{2+} through the paracellular route. The saturable component was most evident in the duodenum, less so in jejunum, was not observable in the ileum of the rat, and decreases with age. These aspects of calcium absorption related to the aging process are discussed in detail by Armbrecht (this volume).

Despite the minimization of the active transport of calcium in the ileum, the earlier experiments of Marcus and Lengemann (1962) clearly showed that most of calcium that is absorbed by the rat (and probably in the human) occurs in the ileum and this due to the long resident time of ingesta in this segment as compared to the duodenum and jejunum.

VITAMIN D METABOLISM AND SOME MOLECULAR EFFECTS

The efficiency of calcium absorption is influenced by diet composition and physiological states. There is an increase in the rate of calcium absorption in animals fed calcium-deficient diets, and this adaptation phenomenon is manifested through alterations in vitamin D metabolism.   Similarly, the efficiency of calcium absorption is greater in growing than in non-growing animals, in pregnant than in non-pregnant mammals, in hens during the egg-laying period, and in lactating in contrast to non-lactating animals. These changes are again manifested through alterations in vitamin D metabolism and point to the central role of vitamin D in the intestinal phase of calcium homeostasis.

Absorbed vitamin D enters the lymph in association with chylomicrons and is rapidly sequestered by the liver (Haddad, 1987). It is in this organ that vitamin D is transformed into the 25-hydroxylated derivative, 25(OH)D or calcidiol. This reaction is not apparently limiting under usual nutritional and physiological conditions.

Vitamin D_3 is also synthesized in the skin by an ultraviolet-light catalyzed reaction from the precursor, 7-dehydrocholesterol.

The 25(OH)D metabolite is the major form of vitamin D in the circulation and the concentration of 25(OH)D in blood is a useful indicator of vitamin D status of an individual.   The 25(OH)D metabolite is further hydroxylated in the 1 or 24 position in the kidney to yield $1,25(OH)_2D$ or $24,25(OH)_2D$. Under conditions of calcium need or calcium deficiency, the synthesis of the $1,25(OH)_2D_3$ predominates. Under conditions of calcium sufficiency or overabundance, the amount of $1,25(OH)_2D_3$ synthesized declines and that of $24,25(OH)_2D_3$ increases, yielding a well-documented reciprocol relationship between these metabolites (DeLuca, 1979; Norman, 1979).   A number of other metabolites of vitamin D_3 have been identified but their physiological significance remains to be defined (DeLuca, 1988; Norman, 1987).

The $1,25(OH)_2D_3$ or calcitriol is the most biologically active metabolite of vitamin D and considered to be the hormonal form. Its synthesis is feed-back controlled, the rate of synthesis affected by parathyroid hormone, phosphate, calcium, $1,25(OH)_2D_3$ per se, and other factors (DeLuca, 1979, 1988; Norman, 1979, 1987). During periods of calcium deficiency, and during growth, pregnancy and lactation, the formation of $1,25(OH)_2D_3$ increases.   In the aging animal, the conversion of 25(OH)D to $1,25(OH)_2D_3$ is less efficient than in the younger animal (Armbrecht et al., 1980) which is apparently reflected in the decreased capacity of the maturer individual to adapt to low calcium intakes (Armbrecht et al.,1979).

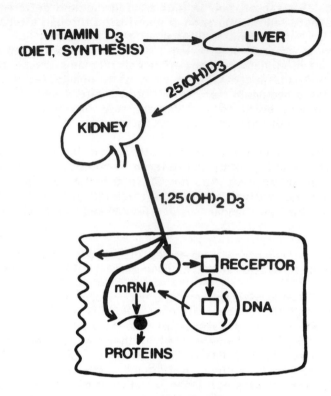

VITAMIN D$_3$
(DIET, SYNTHESIS)

LIVER

25(OH)D$_3$

KIDNEY

1,25(OH)$_2$D$_3$

RECEPTOR

mRNA

DNA

PROTEINS

INTESTINE

Fig. 3.   Proposed Actions of the Vitamin D Hormone on the Intestinal Cell. The vitamin D hormone, 1,25(OH)$_2$D$_3$, is formed by two sequential hydroxylations in the liver and kidney, respectively. Upon entering the enterocyte, 1,25(OH)$_2$D$_3$ binds to a specific receptor that, through interaction with the genomic apparatus, stimulates the synthesis of mRNA's coded for transport proteins, one of which is the vitamin D-induced calcium-binding protein, calbindin-D.   In addition to this transcriptional function of 1,25(OH)$_2$D$_3$, there is also evidence for an effect on translation and a more direct effect on cellular components that increase the permeability of the brush border membrane to Ca^{2+}. These various factors would act in parallel and synergistically to account for the overall effect of vitamin D on calcium transort across the intestinal epithelium.   It might be speculated that specific intracellular receptors for 1,25(OH)$_2$D$_3$ are intermediaries for both the genomic and non-genomic responses of the cell to the vitamin D hormone.

The intracellular $1,25(OH)_2D$ receptor was first identified in the intestine of chicks and since shown to be present in a number of different cell types, including those involved in systemic homeostasis, the kidney and the skeleton (Haussler, 1986). The receptor-$1,25(OH)_2D$ complex is found primarily in the nucleus in association with chromatin and, like other steroids, induces the synthesis of messenger RNA (or RNA's) coded for specific calcium transport proteins (Fig. 3). Thus far, only one protein has been shown to be synthesized de novo by the nuclear action of $1,25(OH)_2D_3$ and that being the vitamin D-induced calcium-binding protein (Wasserman and Fullmer, 1983), now termed calbindin-D. Other proteins and biochemical reactions are also stimulated in the intestine by $1,25(OH)_2D$ and these include the intestinal membrane calcium-binding protein (IMCaI) of Kowarski et al.,(1987) and Kowarski and Schachter (1980), alkaline phosphatase (cf. review of Wasserman and Chandler, 1985, for references) and an actin-like protein (Wilson and Lawson, 1978). However, each of these proteins are present in the severely vitamin D-deficient intestine, and are increased in concentration in response to vitamin D repletion. Further, the activity of various enzymes in addition to alkaline phosphatase are stimulated by vitamin D or $1,25(OH)_2D$ and these include adenylate cyclase (Corradino, 1974; Long et al., 1986) guanylate cyclase (Vesely and Juan, 1984), ornithine decarboxylase (Takahashi et al., 1982), phospholipase A_2 (O'Doherty, 1978) and enzymes involved in phospholipid metabolism (Rasmussen et al., 1982). It is conceivable that the activity of some of these enzymes, and the increased synthetic rate of certain proteins, are indirect consequences of vitamin D due to changes in intracellular Ca^{2+} concentrations.

It is primarily within the cytosolic compartment of the intestinal cell that calbindin-D, a primary $1,25(OH)_2D_3$-induced intestinal gene product, is located (Morrissey et al.,1975; Jande et al, 1981; Thorens et al., 1982; Taylor, 1983; Taylor et al.,1984). Calbindin-D in chick intestine and other tissues and organs of that species has a molecular weight of about 30,000 daltons, binds 4 Ca^{2+} ions per molecular with high affinity ($2 \times 10^6 M^{-1}$) and is an acidic protein (Wasserman and Fullmer, 1983). The calbindin-D present in mammalian intestine is smaller, having a molecular weight of about 10,000 daltons, two high affinity binding sites ($2 \times 10^6 M^{-1}$) and is also an acidic protein (loc cit). The calbindin present in kidney, brain and other organs of mammals has a molecular weight of about 28,000 daltons and is immunologically related but not identical to the avian protein. These calbindins are soluble in aqueous solutions and released from intestinal mucosa by simple homogenization procedures. However, about 5-10% of the protein appears to be tightly associated with membranous and other components of the enterocyte, releasable from these components by detergents, such as Triton X-100 (Feher and Wasserman, 1979; Shimura and Wasserman, 1984).

In vitamin D-replete animals, the calbindins-D are present at relatively high concentrations and within the millimolar range. The estimated concentration of calbindin-D in chick intestine is about 0.3-0.4mM, in the rat about 0.2-0.3mM (Bronner et al., 1986) and, in the pig, about 0.3mM (Vendeland, 1983). The concentration of calbindin within the intestinal cell exceeds that of calmodulin by a factor of about 10.

The quantitative relationship between calbindin and the efficiency or rate of calcium absorption has been examined in several laboratories and a correlation coefficient between these parameters is usually 0.9 or greater (Morrissey and Wasserman, 1971; Bar and Hurwitz, 1972). This close relationship was shown to hold from studies on calcium absorption as a function of aging (Armbrecht et al., 1979; Bronner et al., 1986), as a function of calcium and phosphorus intake (Morrissey and Wasserman, 1971), and as a function of cortisone administration (Feher and Wasserman, 1979a; 1979b). The amount of calcium deposited in the eggshell is also directly related to the calbindin content of the egg shell gland of the uterus of the laying hen (Bar et al., 1984).

The appearance of calbindin-D in the intestinal mucosa of vitamin D-deficient animal after a single dose of $1,25(OH)_2D_3$, or the addition of $1,25(OH)_2D_3$ to embryonic chick intestine in culture, has been shown by some investigators to coincide with a stimulation of calcium transport (Wasserman et al., 1982; Roche et al., 1984, Corradino 1977; Bishop et al., 1983) whereas others have reported that the increase in calcium transport after a pulse of $1,25(OH)_2D_3$ precedes the appearance of calbindin-D (Morrissey et al., 1978; Spencer et al., 1976). These differences might be explained on the basis of different methodologies in measuring calcium absorption and the sensitivity of the calbindin-D assays. In any event, the close quantitative relationship between calbindin and the efficiency of calcium absorption provides reasonable evidence for a significant function of this protein in the epithelial transport of calcium. Bronner et al. (1986) suggest a specific direct relationship between calbindin and the active intestinal transport of calcium from their studies in the rat.

INTESTINAL CALCIUM TRANSPORT:
PHYSIOLOGICAL AND BIOCHEMICAL ASPECTS

The transfer of Ca^{2+} across the intestinal epithelial membrane could occur by three proposed processes of calcium absorption: by the diffusion-active transport model, by movement through the paracellular route and/or by an endocyte-exototic mechanism. Each of these will be briefly discussed in turn.

The Diffusion-Active Transport-Model

This and other models of Ca^{2+} absorption is depicted in Fig. 4, and the diffusion-active transport model is well accepted as the most probable manner by which most Ca^{2+} is absorbed when intraluminal Ca^{2+} concentrations are in the low millimolar range.

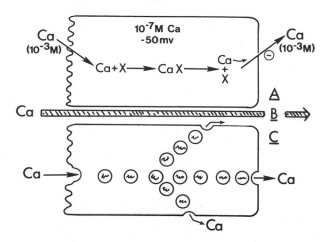

Fig. 4. Processes of the Transfer of Ca^{2+} Across the Intestinal Epithelium. Three models of calcium absorption are depicted. (A) represents the diffusion-active transport model in which Ca^{2+} enters the cell by a downhill diffusional-type process, subsequently diffusing through the cytosol as the free ion and primarily in association with the vitamin D-induced calcium-binding protein, calbindin-D, and extruded up-hill from the cell by energy-dependent processes. (B) depicts the direct transfer of Ca^{2+} from lumen to the interstitial space of the lamina propria via the paracellular path. (C) shows the possible transmural transfer of Ca^{2+} by an endocytotic-exocytotic mechanism (cf. text for discussion and references).

Calcium entry at the brush border   The first step is the transfer of Ca^{2+} across the brush border membrane. Studies by several investigators have demonstrated that the uptake of Ca^{2+} by isolated brush border membrane vesicles is greater in vesicles obtained from vitamin D-replete animals than those from vitamin D-deficient animals (Rasmussen et al., 1979; Bikle et al., 1981). Much of the Ca^{2+} accumulated by the brush border vesicles is bound to components on the inner surface of the membrane (Miller et al, 1982; Wilson and Lawson, 1979). The accelerated uptake of luminal Ca^{2+} by intestinal mucosa was also shown in detailed in vivo studies, using the in situ ligated loop technique (Bikle et al.,1981; Wasserman et al.,1982). Therefore, the rate of entry of Ca^{2+} across the brush border membrane down its gradient is apparently positively affected by vitamin D. The molecular basis of this response is not precisely known but might involve an alteration of the phospholipid and fluidity character of the brush border membrane as originally proposed by Rasmussen et al.(1982). A change in membrane fluidity due to vitamin D was recently confirmed by Brasitus et al.(1986). The IMCal protein identified in rat intestinal brush borders, (Kowarski and Schachter, 1980; Kowarski et al., 1987) and brush border alkaline phosphatase might also be involved in the Ca^{2+} transport reaction at this site.   The concentration of alkaline phosphatase is greater in the brush borders of enterocytes of vitamin D-replete animals than that of vitamin D-deficient animals. However, the time course of its increase after the administration of $1,25(OH)_2D_3$ to vitamin D-deficient animals has tended to relegate it to a secondary role in the vitamin D-mediated calcium absorptive process.

Although total alkaline phosphatase activity does not change detectably shortly after $1,25(OH)_2D_3$ repletion, the molecule is rapidly altered by $1,25(OH)_2D_3$ repletion (Moriuchi and DeLuca, 1975). This $1,25(OH)_2D_3$ dependent isozyme of alkaline phosphatase differs from the native form by the amount of sialic acid associated with it, which could affect its properties, including Ca^{+2} and Mg^{+2} binding. Other evidence for a role of alkaline phosphatase in Ca^{2+} absorption is the direct correlation between these parameters derived from studies on the action of glucocorticoids on Ca^{2+} absorption by the intestine (Feher and Wasserman, 1979a,b).   In addition, alkaline phosphatase activity was shown by Freund (1982) to be increased by the presence of calbindin-D, and Norman and Leathers (1982) reported that photoaffinity-labeled calbindin-D reacted specifically with brush border alkaline phosphatase. Yet, definitive evidence for a role of alkaline phosphatase in Ca^{2+} translocation and is still lacking.

Bikle et al.(1984) and Bikle and Munson (1985) showed that the ubiqitous high affinity calcium-binding protein, calmodulin, is translocated to the brush border region when vitamin D deficient chicks are given $1,25(OH)_2D_3$. Calmodulin prominently binds to the 105 kDa cytoskeletal protein. The function of brush border calmodulin, as suggested by Bikle et al.(loc cit), could be to protect Ca^{2+} sensitive components of cytoskeleton that underly the brush border membrane. We had previously observed that calbindin-D is bound to isolated brush border vesicles and specifically in association with a protein of about 66,000 daltons (Shimura and Wasserman, 1984).

The Ca^{2+} sequestered by binding sites in the brush border membrane might function to control the operation of Ca^{2+} "channels". As the Ca^{2+} concentration increases in the cytosol adjacent to the brush border membrane, the Ca^{2+} influx pathway might close, preventing an excessive amount of luminal Ca^{2+} from entering the cell. In this vein, Taylor and Windhager (1979) proposed that Na^+ entry across the brush border of epithelial cells is controlled by Ca^{2+} sensitive channels. The aqueous channel through the gap junction has long been known to close as the intracellular Ca^{2+} concentration increases (Lowenstein and Rose, 1978).

Transfer of calcium through the cytosol   The vitamin D-dependent transfer of Ca^{2+} through the brush border membrane to the basal lateral membrane is considered to be a function of the vitamin D-induced calbindin-D. The affinity constant of calbindin-D and the high concentration of this protein within the intestinal cell indicate that it is quite suitable to act as a calcium buffer, potentially preventing Ca^{2+} from reaching toxic levels during the course of absorption of calcium. In addition to this buffering function of calbindin-D, it was proposed on theoretical grounds that calbindin-D could facilitate the transfer of Ca^{2+} from the brush border region to the basal lateral membrane (Kretsinger et al.,1982). The basis of this mechanism is that Ca^{2+} can diffuse to the region of the calcium pump as both the free Ca^{2+} ion and calcium bound to calbindin-D. Since the affinity of the Ca pump for Ca^{2+} exceeds that of calbindin-D by a factor of 2-3, the active extrusion of Ca^{2+} across the basal lateral membrane would include both the free diffusible Ca^{2+} and, in addition, Ca^{2+} released from calbindin-D in the region of the Ca pump. Support for calbindin serving as a diffusional facilitator comes from the studies by Feher (1983), using an in vitro three compartment model system.

The Kretsinger-Feher hypothesis of calbindin function predicts that the transfer of Ca^{2+} in the opposite direction, i.e., from plasma (extracellular fluid) to lumen, should also be increased. This was indeed demonstrated several years ago (Wasserman et al.,1966) when it was observed that ^{45}Ca entered the intestinal lumen from blood at a faster rate in vitamin D-replete animals than in vitamin D-deficient animals.

Transfer across the basal-lateral membrane The responsiveness of the calcium pump to vitamin D is an area of uncertainty at the present time. Ghijsen and Van Os (1982) reported that the Ca pump of rat intestine is vitamin D-responsive, as did others (Walters and Weiser, 1987; Chandler et al.,1984). However, vitamin D was considered by Van Corven et al. (1986) to act indirectly by protecting the Ca pump from the deleterious action of proteolytic and lipolytic enzyme. In actuality, the acceleration of overall calcium transport by vitamin D might not require a stimulation of pump activity. In the view of some (Van Os, 1987; Bronner et al.,1986), the Ca pump is normally "starved" for Ca^{2+} and additional Ca^{2+} presented to the pump during the course of vitamin D-stimulated calcium absorption can be readily accommodated.

The Endocytoic-Exocytic Model

The possibility that Ca^{2+} is translocated through the cell in association with lysosomes or as membrane-bound Ca^{2+} packets was proposed a few years ago, based on electron probe analysis (Warner and Coleman, 1975) and histological evidence (Davis et al., 1979; Davis and Jones, 1981). This would provide a way of moving Ca^{2+} through the cell without affecting the resting level of calcium within the cytosol. More recent studies by Nemere et al. (1986) provide biochemical evidence for the existence of a Ca^{2+}-containing vesicular component in the intestinal cell that is apparently $1,25(OH)_2D$ responsive and contains a limited amount of calbindin-D.

According to this model, Ca^{2+} is incorporated into vesicles at the brush border and transported through the cytoplasm in this form, to be released into the extracellular fluid by an exocytotic process at the basal lateral membrane, or coalesces with a lysosome to form a secondary lysosome that in turn releases sequestered calcium in the parenteral direction.

The Paracellular Route

As previously mentioned, the non-saturable component of Ca^{2+} absorption that becomes increasingly evident as intraluminal Ca^{2+} increases is thought to be by diffusion through the paracellular path. Definitive evidence for this path of calcium absorption is virtually non-existent and based primarily on theoretical grounds (Wasserman and Taylor, 1969) and the response of Ca^{2+} translocation across the intestine to applied transcellular voltages,using in vitro preparations (Nellans and Kimberg, 1978). The latter approach provided evidence for the electrophoretic transfer of Ca^{2+} across the epithelial cell layer, presumably through the paracellular route.

GENOMIC AND NON-GENOMIC THEORIES OF VITAMIN D ACTION

The genomic theory of vitamin D action had earlier support from the temporal lag period between vitamin D or $1,25(OH)_2D_3$ administration to vitamin D-depleted animals and the resultant physiological response. The lag period represented the time required for the vitamin D hormone to associate with the receptor, for the transfer of the $1,25(OH)_2D_3$ receptor complex to the nucleus, the synthesis of the appropriate mRNA, and then the ribosomal synthesis of the gene product. The lag period after vitamin D administration is about 12-16 hrs and after $1,25(OH)_2D_3$ administration, 4-6 hr. However, the response time to $1,25(OH)_2D_3$ is considerably shortened if $1,25(OH)_2D_3$ is administered to vitamin D replete animals. Bronner and Buckley (1982) advanced the notion that $1,25(OH)_2D_3$ increases calbindin-D concentrations rapidly in vitamin D-replete animals by a post-translational mechanism (Fig. 4). Bikle et al,(1981) showed that Ca^{2+} uptake into the enterocyte occurred relatively soon after the $1,25(OH)_2D_3$ administration to rachitic chicks and presumably before protein synthesis took place.

An extremely rapid response of the intestinal absorptive process to $1,25(OH)_2D_3$ was demonstrated by Nemere and Norman (1984), using an in vitro intestinal and vascular perfusion system in the chick. The addition of $1,25(OH)_2D_3$ to the circulatory system increased Ca^{2+} absorption in a matter of minutes; however, this rapid response occurred only in vitamin D-replete animals. The vitamin D-deficient animal does not respond. In the same model, parathyroid hormone (PTH) also yielded a very rapid increase in calcium absorption and again only in vitamin D-replete animals (Nemere and Norman, 1986). The parathyroid hormone effect is unexpected since previous studies suggested that the primary (or only) role of PTH in calcium absorption was indirect, increasing the synthesis of $1,25(OH)_2D_3$ by the renal 1α-hydroxylase system. PTH, in other systems, is known to increase adenylate cyclase activity and $1,25(OH)_2D_3$, directly or indirectly, also stimulates adenylate cyclase as well as guanylate cyclase activity, as previously mentioned. It is conceivable that the rapid effect of $1,25(OH)_2D_3$ in vitamin D-replete animals is due to protein kinase activation by cAMP and/or cGMP, and possibly by Ca^{2+} itself.

REFERENCES

Ammann P, Rizzoli R, Fleisch H (1986). Calcium absorption in rat large intestine in vivo: availability of dietary calcium. Am J Physiol 251:G14-8.

Armbrecht HJ, Zenser TV, Davis BB (1980). Effect of age on the conversion of 25-hydroxyvitamin D_3 to 1,25-dihydroxyvitamin D_3 by kidney of rat. J Clin Invest 66:1118-1123.

Armbrecht HJ, Zenser TV, Bruns ME, Davis BB (1979). Effect of age on intestinal calcium absorption and adaptation to dietary calcium. Am J Physiol 236:769-774.

Bar A, Hurwitz S (1972). Relationship of duodenal calcium-binding protein to calcium absorption in the laying fowl. Comp Biochem Physiol 41:735-744.

Bar A, Rosenberg J, Hurwitz S (1984). The lack of relationships between vitamin D_3 metabolites and calcium-binding protein in the eggshell gland of laying hens. Comp Biochem Physiol 788:75-79.

Berridge MJ, Irvine RF (1984). Inositol trisphosphate, a novel second messenger system in cellular signal transduction. Nature 312:315-321.

Bikle DD, Munson S (1985). 1,25-Dihydroxyvitamin D increases calmodulin binding to specific proteins in the chick duodenal brush border membrane. J Clin Invest 76:2312-2316.

Bikle DD, Munson S, Chafouleas J (1984). Calmodulin may mediate 1,25-dihydroxyvitamin D-stimulated intestinal calcium transport. FEBS Lett 174:30-33.

Bikle DD, Morrissey RL, Zolock DT, Rasmussen H (1981). The intestinal response to vitamin D. Rev Physiol Biochem Pharmacol 89:63-142.

Bishop CW, Kendrick NC, DeLuca HF (1983). Induction of calcium-binding protein before 1,25-dihydroxyvitamin D_3 stimulation of duodenal calcium uptake. J Biol Chem 258:1305-1310.

Brasitus TA, Dudeja PK, Eby B, Lau K (1986). Correction by 1,25-dihydroxycholecalciferol of the abnormal fluidity and lipid composition of enterocyte brush border membranes in vitamin Ddeprived rats. J Biol Chem 261:16404-16409.

Bronner F, Pansu D, Stein WD (1986). An analysis of intestinal calcium transport across the rat intestine. Am J Physiol 250: G561-9.

Bronner F, Buckley M (1982). The molecular nature of 1,25-(OH)$_2$D$_3$ -induced calcium-binding protein biosynthesis in the rat. Adv Exp Med Biol 151:355-360.

Chandler JS, Meyer SA, Wasserman RH (1984). Effects of 1,25-dihydroxycholecalciferol on the chick intestinal basolateral calcium pump. Fed Proc 43:485.

Corradino RA (1974) Embryonic chick intestine in organ culture: interaction of adenylate cyclase system and vitamin D$_3$-mediated calcium absorptive mechanism. Endocrinology 94:1607-1614.

Corradino RA (1977). Cyclic AMP regulation of the 1$^\alpha$,25-(OH)$_2$D$_3$-mediated intestinal calcium absorptive mechanism. In Norman AW, Schaefer K, Coburn JW, DeLuca HF, Fraser D, Grigoleit HG, v. Herrath D (eds), "Vitamin D. Biochemical, Chemical and Clinical Aspects Related to Calcium Metabolism" Berlin, de Gruyter, pp 231-240.

Corradino RA, Wasserman RH (1971). Vitamin D$_3$: induction of calcium-binding protein in embryonic chick intestine in vitro. Science 172:731-733.

Davis WL, Jones RG, Hagler HK (1979). Calcium containing lysosomes in the normal chick duodenum: a histochemical and analytical electron microscopic study. Tissue and Cell 11:127-138.

Davis WL, Jones RG (1981) Early actions of parathyroid hormone and 1,25-dihydroxycholecalciferol on isolated epithelial cells from rat intestine. I. Limited lysosomal enzyme release and calcium uptake. Endocrinology 108:1450-1462.

DeLuca HF (1979). "Vitamin D: Metabolism and Function", Berlin, Springer-Verlag.

DeLuca HF (1988). The vitamin D story: a collaborative effort of basic science and clinical medicine. FASEB J 2:224-36.

Favus MJ, Backman EA (1985). Effects of 1,25(OH)$_2$D$_3$ and calcium channel blockers on cecal calcium transport in the rat. Am J Physiol 248:G676-81.

Favus MJ, Langman CB (1984). Effects of 1,25-dihydroxyvitamin and normal rats. Am J Physiol 246:G268-73.

Feher JJ (1983). Facilitated calcium diffusion by intestinal calcium-binding protein. Am J Physiol 244:303-307.

Feher JJ, Wasserman RH (1978). Evidence for a membrane-bound fraction of chick intestinal calcium-binding protein. Biochim Biophys Acta 540:134-143.

Feher JJ, Wasserman RH (1979a). Intestinal calcium-binding protein and calcium absorption in cortisol-treated chicks: Effects of vitamin D_3 and 1,25-dihydroxyvitamin D_3. Endocrinology 104:547-551.

Feher JJ, Wasserman RH (1979b). Calcium absorption and intestinal calcium-binding protein: quantitative relationship. Am J Physiol 236:556-561.

Freund TS (1982). Vitamin D-dependent intestinal calcium binding protein as an enzyme modulator. In Norman AW, Schaefer K, v. Herrath D, Grigoleit HG (eds), "Vitamin D. Chemical, Biochemical and Clinical Endocrinology of Calcium Metabolism", Berlin, de Gruyter, pp 249-251.

Freund T, Bronner F (1975). Stimulation in vitro by 1,25-dihydroxyvitamin D_3 of intestinal cell calcium uptake and calcium-binding protein. Science 190:1300-1302.

Ghijsen WEJM, Van Os CH (1982). 1,25-Dihydroxyvitamin D_3 regulates ATP-dependent calcium transport in basolateral plasma membranes of rat enterocytes. Biochim Biophys Acta 689:170-172.

Grinstead WC, Pak CY, Krejs GJ (1984). Effect of 1,25-dihydroxyvitamin D_3 on calcium absorption in the colon of healthy humans. Am J Physiol 247:G189-92.

Haddad JG (1987). Traffic, binding and cellular access of vitamin D sterols. In Peck WA (ed): "Bone and Mineral Research/5", Amsterdam, Elsevier, Vol.5: pp 281-308.

Harrison HE, Harrison HC (1960). Transfer of Ca^{45} across intestinal wall in vitro in relation to the action of vitamin D and cortisol. Am J Physiol 199:265-271.

Haussler M, Nagode LA, Rasmussen H (1970). Induction of intestinal brush border alkaline phosphatase by vitamin D and identity with Ca-ATPase. Nature 228:1199-1201.

Haussler MR (1986). Vitamin D receptors: nature and function. Annu Rev Nutr 6:527-562.

Jande SS, Tolnai S, Lawson DE (1981). Immunohistochemical localization of vitamin D-dependent calcium-binding protein in duodenum, kidney, uterus and cerebellum of chickens. Histochemistry 71:99-116.

Kowarski S, Cowen LA, Takahashi MT, Schachter D (1987). Tissue distribution and vitamin D dependence of IMCAL in the rat. Am J Physiol 253:G411-9.

Kowarski S, Schachter D (1980). Intestinal membrane calcium-binding protein. Vitamin D-dependent membrane component of the intestinal calcium transport mechanism. J Biol Chem 255:10834-10840.

Kretsinger RH, Mann JE, Simmons JB (1982). Model of the

facilitated diffusion of calcium by the intestinal calcium binding proteins. In Norman AW, Schaefer K, Herrath DV, Gregoleit H-G (eds), "Vitamin D. Chemical, Biochemical and Clinical Endocrinology of Calcium Metabolism" Berlin, de Gruyter, pp 233-248.

Lowenstein WR, Rose B (1978). Calcium in (junctional) intercellular communications and a thought on its behavior in intracellular communication. An NY Acad Sci 307:285-307.

Long RG, Bikle DD, Munson SJ (1986). Stimulation by 1,25-dihydroxyvitamin D_3 of adenylate cyclase along the villus of chick duodenum. Endocrinology 119:2568-2573.

Marcus CS, Lengemann FW (1962). Absorption of Ca^{45} and Se^{85} from solid and liquid food at various levels of the alimentary tract of the rat. J Nutr 77:155-160.

Miller A 3d, Li ST, Bronner F (1982). Characterization of calcium binding to brush-border membranes from rat duodenum. Biochem J 208:773-781.

Moriuchi S, DeLuca HF (1975). The effect of vitamin D_3 metabolites on membrane proteins of chick duodenal brush borders. Arch Biochem Biophys 174:367-372.

Morrissey RL, Bucci TJ, Richard B, Empson N, Lufkin EG (1975). Calcium-binding protein: its cellular localization in jejunum, kidney and pancreas. Proc Soc Exp Biol Med 149:56-60.

Morrissey RL, Empson RN, Zolock DT, Bikle DD, Bucci TJ (1978). Intestinal response to 1α, 25-dihydroxycholecalciferol II. A timed study. BBA 538:34-41.

Morrissey RL, Wasserman RH (1971). Calcium absorption and calcium-binding protein in chicks on differing calcium and phosphorus intakes. Am J Physiol 220:1509-1515.

Nellans HN, Kimberg DV (1978). Cellular and paracellular calcium transport in rat ileum: Effects of dietary calcium. Am J Physiol 236:E726-E737.

Nemere I, Norman AW (1984). Parathyroid hormone stimulates calcium transport in perfused duodena from normal chicks: Comparison with the rapid (transcaltochic) effect of 1,25-dihydroxyvitamin D_3. Endocrinol. 119:1406-1408.

Nemere I, Norman AW (1986). Rapid action of 1,25-dihydroxyvitamin D_3 on calcium transport in perfused chick duodenum. Effect of inhibitors. J Bone Min Res 2:99-107.

Nemere I, Leathers W, Norman AW (1986). 1,25-Dihydroxyvitamin D_3-mediated intestinal calcium transport Biochemical identification of lysosomes containing calcium and calcium-binding Protein (calbindin-D_{28K}). J Biol Chem 261:16106-16114.

Nishizuka Y (1986). Studies and perspectives of protein kinase C. Science 233:305-312.

Norman AW (1979)."Vitamin D: The Calcium Homeostasic Steroid Hormone", New York, Academic Press.

Norman AW (1987). Studies on the vitamin D endocrine system in the avian. J Nutr 117:797-807.

Norman AW, Leathers V (1982). Preparation of a photoaffinity probe for the vitamin D-dependent intestinal calcium binding protein: evidence for a calcium dependent, specific interaction with intestinal alkaline phosphatase. Biochem Biophys Res Commun 108:220-226.

O'Doherty PJA (1978) . 1,25-Dihydroxyvitamin D_3 increases the activity of the intestinal phosphatidycholine deacylation-reacylation cycle. Lipids 14:75-77.

Pansu D, Bellaton C, Roche C, Bronner F (1983). Duodenal and ileal calcium absorption in the rat and effects of vitamn D. Am J Physiol 244:695-700.

Pansu D, Bellaton C, Bronner F (1981). Effect of Ca intake on saturable and nonsaturable components of duodenal Ca transport. Am J Physiol 240:32-37.

Rasmussen H (1986). The calcium messenger system. N Engl J Med 314:1094-1101, 1164-1170.

Rasmussen H, Fontaine O, Max EE, Goodman DBP (1979). The effect of 1α-hydroxyvitamin D_3 administration on calcium transport in chick intestine brush border membrane vesicles. J Biol Chem 254:2993-2999.

Rasmussen H, Matsumoto T, Fontaine O, Goodman DB (1982). Role of changes in membrane lipid structure in the action of 1,25-dihydroxyvitamin D_3. Fed Proc 41:72-77.

Rega AF (1985). The measurement of Ca^{2+} in the cytosol. In Rega AF, Garrahan PJ (eds): "The Ca^{2+} Pump of Plasma Membranes:, Boca Raton, FL, CRC Press, pp 1-11.

Roche C, Bellaton C, Pansu D, Bronner F (1984). Simultaneous induction of CaBP and active calcium transport in rat duodenum by 1,25-dihydroxyvitamin D_3. Prog Clin Biol Res 168:267-271.

Schachter D, Rosen SM (1959). Active transport of Ca^{45} by the small intestine and its dependence on vitamin D. Am J Physiol 196:357-362.

Shimura F, Wasserman RH (1984). Membrane-associated vitamin D-induced calcium-binding protein (CaBP): quantification by a radioimmunoassay and evidence for a specific CaBP in purified intestinal brush borders. Endocrinology 115:1964-1972.

Spencer R, Charman M, Wilson P, Lawson E (1976). Vitamin D-stimulated intestinal calcium absorption may not involve calcium-binding protein directly. Nature 263:161-163.

Takahashi N, Shinki T, Kawate N, Samejima K, Nishii Y, Suda T (1982). Distribution of ornithine decarboxylase activity induced by 1α,25-dihydroxyvitamin D3 in chick duodenal villus mucosa. Endocrinology 111:1539-1545.

Taylor AN, Gleason WA Jr, Lankford GK (1984). Immunocytochemical localization of rat intestinal vitamin D-dependent calcium-binding protein. J Histochem Cytochem 32:153-158.

Taylor AN (1983). Intestinal vitamin D-induced calcium-binding protein: time-course of immunocytological localization following 1,25-dihydroxyvitamin D3. J Histochem Cytochem 31:426-432.

Taylor AN, Windhager EE (1979). Possible role of cytocolic calcium and Na-Ca exchange in regulation of transepithelial sodium transport. Am J Physiol 236:F505-F512.

Thorens B, Roth J, Norman AW, Perrelet A, Orci L (1982). Immunocytochemical localization of the vitamin D-dependent calcium binding protein in chick duodenum. J Cell Biol 94:115-122.

Toverud SU, Dostal LA (1986). Calcium absorption during development: experimental studies of the rat small intestine. J Pediatr Gastroenterol Nutr 5:688-695.

Van Corven EJJM, DeJong MD, Van Os CH (1986). Enterocyte isolation procedure specifically affects ATP-dependent Ca^{2+}-transport in small intestine plasma membranes. Cell Calcium 7:89-99.

Van Os CH (1987). Transcellular calcium transport in intestinal and renal epithelial cells. Biochim Biophys Acta 906:195-222.

Vendeland SC (1983). Adaptation of pigs to a calcium-deficient diet; Alteration of intestinal components. Thesis.

Vesely DL, Juan D (1984). Cation-dependent vitamin D activation of human renal cortical quanylate cyclase. Am J Physiol 246:E115-20.

Walters JR, Weiser MM (1987). Calcium transport by rat duodenal villus and crypt basolateral membranes. Am J Physiol 252:G170-177.

Warner RR, Coleman JR (1975). Electron probe analysis of calcium transport by small intestine. J Cell Biol 64:54-74.

Wasserman RH, Chandler JS (1985). Molecular mechanisms of intestinal calcium absorption. In Peck WA (ed) "Bone and Mineral Research/3", Amsterdam, Elsevier, vol. 3, pp 181-211.

Wasserman RH, Fullmer CS (1983). Calcium transport proteins, calcium absorption, and vitamin D. Annu Rev Physiol 45:375-390.

Wasserman RH, Brindak ME, Meyer SA, Fullmer CS (1982). Evidence for multiple effects of vitamin D3 on calcium absorption: response of rachitic chicks, with or without partial vitamin D3 repletion, to 1,25-dihydroxyvitamin D3. Proc Natl Acad Sci USA

79:7939-7943.

Wasserman RH, Kallfelz FA, Comar CL (1961). Active transport of calcium by rat duodenum in vivo. Science 133:883-884.

Wasserman RH, Kallfelz FA. (1962). Vitamin D3 and the unidirectional calcium fluxes across the rachitic chick duodenum. Am J Physiol 203:221-224, 1962.

Wasserman RH, Taylor AN (1969). Some aspects of the intestinal absorption of calcium, with special reference to vitamin D. In Comar CL, Bronner F (eds) "Mineral Metabolism, An Advanced Treatise" New York: Academic Press, pp 321-403.

Wasserman RH, Taylor AN, Kallfelz FA (1966). Vitamin D and transfer of plasma calcium to intestinal lumen in chicks and rats. Am J Physiol 211:419-423.

Williamson JR, Cooper RH, Joseph SK, Thomas AP (1985). Inositol trisphosphate and diacylglycerol as intracellular second messengers in liver. Am J Physiol 248:C203-C216.

Wilson PW, Lawson DEM (1978). Incorporation of ^{3}H leucine into an actin-like protein in response to 1,25-dihydroxycholecalciferol in chick intestinal brush borders. Biochem J 173:627-631.

Wilson PW, and Lawson DEM (1979). Calcium binding activity by chick intestinal brush-border membrane vesicles. Pflugers Arch 389:69-74.

Mineral Homeostasis in the Elderly, pages 35–68
© *1989 Alan R. Liss, Inc.*

TRACE METAL ABSORPTION IN THE AGED

Noel W. Solomons, M.D.

Center for Studies of Sensory Impairment, Aging
and Metabolism, the research branch of the National Committee for the Blind and Deaf of Guatemala, Guatemala City, Guatemala.

NUTRITION OF THE AGED POPULATION

Throughout the life-span, the organism requires new
supplies of nutrients and adequate and appropriate reserves
of the same for metabolic and structural purposes. As the
population ages, and that segment beyond 65 years of age
expands, increasing attention is being focused on nutrition
and aging. As we direct that attention, we find a blanket
of ignorance regarding such issues as the specific dietary
requirements for the elderly and the state of nutritional
health of the very old. This situation derives in part from
historical factors such as the fact that the Recommended
Dietary Allowances (NAS, 1980) of the Food and Nutrition
Board of the National Academy of Sciences has lumped adult
requirements after 51 years of age, and the fact that the
National Health and Nutrition Examination Surveys (NHANES I
& II) only included persons up to age 74 years. These deficiencies in our understanding are apparently being redressed
somewhat belatedly: 1) The United States Department of Agriculture's Human Nutrition Research Center on Aging in Boston
has a specific mandate to refine our estimates of individual
nutrient intake requirements; and 2) it was recommended in
the planning for NHANES III that the elderly up to 85 years
be included.

Our concern for nutrition and aging spans -- and must
span -- a continuum from fundamental questions of aging biology to applied issues of how we respond to the nutritional
needs of an increasingly sizeable aged population. Hence,

any review of a topic such as "The Impact of Aging on Trace
Mineral Absorption" must relate itself to all degrees of the
spectrum. As huge gaps exist in our understanding of the
theme, it is not surprising that many specific details are
unavailable and unattainable. Specifically with regard to
research in elderly human subjects, or even with experimental animal aging model, empirical data are at a premium.
Irv Rosenberg and I edited a 314 page book, *Absorption and
Malabsorption of Mineral Nutrients* in 1984, a textbook that
covered both macro and trace minerals; a total of 76 lines
of text, equivalent to two pages of text, were devoted to the
changes in mineral absorption that accompany human aging or
the infirmities of the aged. In the present chapter, we
shall make use of *findings* both from experimental animals
and human/clinical literature, and *speculations* and *deduc-
tions* based on insights from various diverse areas. Never
is the reality of generating more questions than answers
more apparent than when we treat issues of the elderly and
of aging.

ABSORPTION AND NUTRITION

Absorption is the process by which molecules and atoms
from the environment enter the interior of the organism via
passage across (or around) the lining cells of the gastrointestinal tract. Absorption can occur all the way from the
stomach to the rectum, although the *small intestine* is the
organ most importantly involved in absorption.

Transport across the gastrointestinal epithelium involves the uptake of *nutrients* (substances essential to the
biological functions), *non-nutrients* (substances that have
no known biological roles, and which occasionally could be
toxic), and *drugs* (substances with "medicinal" or "pharmacological" properties). Parenthetically, the trace metals are
represented in all three categories. The most important
class of absorbed substances, however, are nutrients, and,
in the review, it is important that the process not be taken
out of broad context, and viewed in isolation. Thus, we are
talking about the ability of the aging gut to sustain and
regulate the *nutritional status* of the aging host. The bot-
tom line of our absorption and aging balance-sheet is the
nutriture of the elderly person.

It should be borne in mind, however, that other important processes, namely *retention* and *excretion* of the absorbed nutrient, also influence and determine nutritional
status. To the extent that the elimination of the nutrient
involves the gastrointestinal tract, we shall examine the
effect of aging as well. In summary, the primary purpose of
absorption is to provide nutrients from the diet for metabolic and structural roles in the body. Impaired absorption
has potential consequences for the nutrient status of the
body. Other mechanisms, however, i.e. excretion/retention,
utilization rates, also contribute to the overall nutritional state.

AGING AND GASTROINTESTINAL FUNCTION

Implicit in the topic under discussion is the notion
that advancing years will influence gastrointestinal function in ways that will alter the uptake of trace elements
from the diet. Several reviews on the relationship of aging
and gastrointestinal function have appeared (Bowman and
Rosenberg 1983; Geokas et al., 1985; Steinheber, 1985; Thomson and Keelan, 1986). Two aspects of aging must be considered. The first is normal aging. What are the intrinsic
changes of senescence on human tissues and organs? What
dietary alterations are common in aged populations? The
latter consideration has implications for the *biological
availability*. The second is the *pathological* aspect, that
is, the abnormal (disease) changes that are more frequent --
but not universal or inevitable -- in the aged. This involves both the metabolical, physiological and anatomical
alterations of disease. It also includes the effects of
medications that may be prescribed for degenerative conditions. These drugs may alter the bioavailability of dietary
trace metals.

In general, both the digestive processes for intraluminal and membrane-level hydrolysis of foodstuffs, and the absorptive process for the transcellular uptake of nutrients
have up to a ten-fold excess capacity in adult life. Normal
senescence causes a reduction in most physiological functions
(Shock et al., 1984). Applying these principles, absorptive
capacity will also have declined by some average figure by
the time a person reaches 65 years. This would still leave
the typical elder with considerable reserve capacity. This
is the concept of *average* figures, however. At any given

age, the population would have a considerable *distribution around its mean*. As the function for the group as a whole declines, more and more persons at the lower end of the distribution may pass beyond a threshold at which the function no longer satisfies the needs of that individual.

Absorptive efficiency for many nutrients, notably iron, calcium, and zinc, is governed by feed-back regulation. When the body stores are too low, the intestine *up*-regulates the avidity with which the intestine takes up the nutrient. When the body reserves are adequate or increased, the gut *down*-regulates the nutrient's uptake. At a molecular level, this regulation can be expressed by the control of intraluminal binding ligands, cell surface receptors, intracellular carrier proteins, intracellular storage proteins, or the energetics of transmembrane transport. Any failure of the former response brought about by aging would contribute to depletion. Equally possible in aging would be the failure of the downregulation response allowing *hyper*-absorption of a given nutrient, and this excessive uptake could lead to total-body overload and toxic accumulation in tissues. Thus, senescence of the gastrointestinal tract could alter hydrolytic and transport capacity, and the regulatory control of absorption.

Other changes of the elderly population relate to their behavior in *dietary* selection and intake. Given more sedentary life-styles, total food intake goes down with advancing age. Whether stereotype or common reality, tea and toast are associated with the elderly's diet. Tea contains polyphenolic substances (tannins) in abundance. Dental and peridontal degeneration leads to progressive masticatory failure and certain foods, such as cooked red meats and crisp, hard vegetables become more difficult to negotiate. Moreover, senior citizens are often told to reduce their intake of foods containing animal fat and cholesterol, to diminish the intake of salt, and to increase their intake of calcium either with dairy products or calcium supplements. Since the mid-1970s, a number of claims for beneficial effects of dietary fiber have been reported (Trowell, 1978); these may have encouraged some elderly to increase their fiber consumption.

The composition of foods and beverages determine the chemical form of a nutrient. The chemical form of the nutrient, in turn, is often of importance in the absorption of a mineral. In many solid foods, elements are not free, but firmly bound in the food matrix. They can be in covalent association with a protein, as in metalloenzymes, or in electrochemical chelation arrangements to a non-specific binder. Thus, the dietary prescription to increase intake of calcium, or fiber, or the increased consumption of tea could all alter the absorption of trace elements.

Chronic disease plays an increasing role in life of the elderly. Gastrointestinal disease such as chronic intestinal ischemia, intestinal lymphoma, and pernicious anemia could have direct effects on their digestive and absorptive capacity. Other degenerative diseases such as cardiovascular problems, arthritis and prostatitis call forth the prescription of various drugs and medication. Among the pharmacological agents commonly used by elderly, and potentially influential in metal absorption are: antacids; steroids; antibiotics; and megadoses of nutrients. Ascorbic acid (vitamin C) has become popular in amounts beyond the recognized nutritional requirements. It may influence the absorption of iron and copper. A recent review (Solomons, Ruz, Castillo-Duran, 1988) revealed that oral zinc has been advocated by some for the treatment of prostatitis, arthritis, and smell and taste abnormalities, not to mention dementias and depressive illness. Thus, the pathological -- as well as the senescent -- consequences of advanced age are implicated in alteration of trace metal absorption.

TRACE ELEMENT NUTRIENTS

The trace elements are those elements that constitute 0.01% of body weight (Mertz, 1981), or less of total of 7 g in a 70 kg man. Among trace elements are substances which can be potentially toxic, such as mercury, cadmium, lead, and arsenic, and metals such as rhodium and rubidium which are neither essential nor harmful. Based on observations in mammalian species, we consider that a total of 13 trace elements are "nutrients", that is, they have an important -- if not essential -- role in maintaining health; these include: iron, zinc, copper, manganese, selenium, chromium, cobalt, molybdenum, vanadium, nickel, lithium, iodine and fluorine.

The importance of trace elements in livestock husbandry has been appreciated for many decades (Underwood, 1956), but only in the last 20 years has the role of the substance in human nutrition and metabolism. Even less information on trace elements *specifically related to the elderly or the aging process* is available. From rudimentary and fragmentary findings, however, we have indications that trace elements may play specific and unique roles for the elderly. For instance, zinc at levels above the customary nutritional requirements has been shown to enhance immune function of "healthy and well-nourished" elders (Duchateau et al., 1981; Wagner et al., 1983). Much has been speculated regarding the role of oxidation as a propagator of the aging process reactions (Harman, 1961) and the level of tissue iron may be a determinant of overall oxidative damage. On the antioxidant side of the equation, selenium is an essential component of the antioxidant enzyme, glutathione peroxidase (Levander, 1988), and circulating ceruloplasmin may serve as a free-radical scavenger (Goldstein et al., 1979).

IRON ABSORPTION IN THE AGED

Biology of Iron

Iron is a constituent of a number of proteins in the body. The most important iron metalloproteins, both in abundance and in function, are hemoglobin (or red blood cells) and myoglobin (in skeletal muscle). The principle function of hemoglobin is the transport of oxygen from lungs to tissues. A number of iron-containing enzymes are also found in tissues. Dependencies of various physiological functions on iron leads to non-hematological manifestations of iron deficiency (Jacobs, 1977; Oski, 1985).

The average adult man has 4 g of iron in the body. At any given time, about three grams are contained in nascent and circulating red cells or in tissue enzymes. One gram is distributed in storage compartments (iron reserves), with a third in the liver, a third in skeletal muscle, and a third in the bone marrow and reticuloendothelial systems.

Iron is transported in the circulation in transferrin. Since certain pathogenic micro-organisms have a high requirement for iron, a certain increased susceptibility to bacterial and protozoal infections can arise with iron sufficiency and in iron overload states.

Pertinent Aspects of Iron Absorption

Iron is the third most abundant element on the earth,
and it would seem logical that its *excess* would be more prevalent than its deficiency. The special intestinal mechanism for the uptake of iron may be primarily geared to ex-
cluding an excess accumulation of this metal in our bodies.
In any event, a very complex array of control mechanisms are
in place to govern the intestinal uptake of iron. Dietary
iron is absorbed primarily from the duodenum and upper jejunum, once liberated from its food matrices. Two distinct
dietary forms of iron are recognized by the intestine: 1)
non-heme iron, the *inorganic* salt forms that can be either
divalent and reduced (*ferrous*) or trivalent and oxidized
(*ferric*); 2) *heme* iron, an organic form in the porphyrin
(heme) component of hemoglobin and myoglobin in red meats,
fish and poultry (Lynch, 1984). The latter form is absorbed
as part of the mucosal uptake of the heme ring, and the
elemental iron is only liberated once the moiety is inside
the enterocyte. Absorption of heme iron is relatively unaffected by intraluminal factors. Inorganic iron, on the
other hand, is relatively poorly absorbed. It is most absorbable in its soluble form as the ferrous ion. Ascorbic
acid, meat and gastric acid all tend to favor the solubility
and absorbability of non-heme iron. A large number of dietary factors such as tea, coffee, eggs, and fiber, tend to
bind inorganic iron and render it less bioavailable for uptake by the intestine (Lynch, 1984). For both forms of iron,
a strong, homeostatic regulation is exercised in the transfer to the body. The efficiency of passage of mucosal iron
to the body is inversely related to the iron reserves in the
body. Refsum and Schreiner (1984) have recently suggested
that the macrophages in the intestinal wall may play a cru-
cial role in the regulatory control of iron uptake into the
human body.

Changes in Iron Absorption with Age

So complex are the absorptive processes, one would ex-
pect it to have a number of points of vulnerability to the
aging process. Iron absorption, however, in the elderly is
probably influenced first and foremost by senile, and/or

pathological changes in the stomach. A diminution in the acid secretory capacity occurs in the normal course of aging, producing a relative hypochlorhydria (Bender, 1968). Achlorhydria occurs in a substantial fraction of the elderly (Bhanthumnavin and Schuster, 1977). Since an acid pH favors the solubility of inorganic iron in the intestinal tract, the reduction in acid output that accompanies aging, can be expected to make dietary inorganic iron less available for absorption.

The metabolic balance format has been used to study apparent absorption of iron in six elderly men in the inpatient metabolic unit at the University of California at Berkeley (Turnlund et al., 1981; 1982a; 1988). Subjects consumed a formula diet with 10 mg of iron as ferric chloride, reduced with dilute hydrochloric acid. The authors point out, honestly, the types and magnitudes of errors -- in collections, in analyses of biological materials -- that could affect the results for this or any trace constituent. Their subjects were healthy elderly men, aged 65 to 74 years, confined to the unit for 12 weeks. They underwent adaptation and two 21-day balance periods. Four subjects participated during period #1, and all six were involved in metabolic period #2. Unfortunately, the authors did not report the data on intake and fecal output in a disaggregated manner, so that individual apparent absorption values cannot be computed. Only mean (measured) intake and mean fecal output data for the whole groups by metabolic periods are reported. As shown in Table 1, *on average* the elderly men were close to equilibrium in their intestinal handling of iron (not considering urinary and other insensible losses) (Turnlund et al., 1981). The authors do provide individual iron *retention* data; among subjects and between periods, there was considerable individual variability, with some being more positive and others more negative. Two important interpretative issues, however, are: 1) the relative insensitivity of metabolic balances to *fine* adjustments due to relatively large measurement errors; and 2) the large component of fecal iron from endogenous sources. These combine to make any approximation of *true* absorption impossible.

In the same experiments, however, absorption of a tracer dose of a stable isotope of iron (^{54}Fe) was also given (Turnlund et al., 1982a; 1988). Knowing the level of isotopic enrichment in the diet, and by analyzing the fecal samples from balance collections by thermal ionization mass

TABLE 1. Apparent Absorption of Iron in Six Healthy
Elderly Subjects in the Berkeley Study

Metabolic Period	Mean Dietary Intake (mg/day)	Mean Fecal Excretion (mg/day)	Difference of Means (mg/day)
1	10.0 ± 0.0	9.87 ± 0.29	+ 0.13
2	10.0 ± 0.0	10.40 ± 0.16	− 0.40

Modified after Turnlund et al. (1981).

spectrometry, an estimate for the *fractional absorption* of
the marker is possible. It is the assumption in extrinsic
tagging of meals, that the tracer forms a common pool with
the intrinsic mineral in the diet. Averaged over both metabolic periods, the overall fractional absorption of isotopic
iron was 7.9 ± 2.5% (± SEM). In six healthy young men, aged
22 to 30 years, studied under identical conditions, fractional absorption was 8.0 and 8.2%, respectively, during two balance periods (Turnlund et al., 1988). This represented 0.8
mg of dietary iron absorbed daily by both groups. No differences in iron uptake from the semi-synthetic formula diet
was effected by aging in these healthy male subjects.

The artificial nature of the formula diet should be
emphasized in the interpretation of the Berkeley study, and
any extrapolations to real mixed diets is tentative, and potential unreliable. Moreover, if we examine the results of
the elderly males at the extremes of the distribution, who
consistently had a negative intestinal loss of 0.4 mg daily,
we could calculate that it would take 25000 days (or 8 years)
for them to deplete the normal complement of 1 g of storage
iron in the adult body.

Another perspective on iron absorption and aging --
more from the intestinal physiological than from the dietary perspective -- can be found in a small literature on
intestinal iron absorption involving aqueous trace doses of
radioactive isotopes of iron (^{59}Fe) and either fecal monitoring or whole-body counting. In the original study at the
Home for the Jewish Aged, in Philadelphia in 1963, Frieman

et al. (1963), studied 25 healthy female residents, aged 70
and 79 y, 10 healthy women aged 80 to 87 y, and 9 elderly
men aged 69 to 85 y, for a total of 44 geriatric subjects.
Sixteen healthy younger adults, aged 24 to 60 y, served as
controls (gender distribution not reported). Fecal monitoring for disappearance of a 5 uCi oral dose of ^{59}Fe, given
without carrier iron and without ascorbic acid, was the
method of assessing fractional absorption. Stools were collected for 7 days after dosing. No differences in fractional iron absorption between the older and younger elderly
women, 61 ± 24% versus 57 ± 24% (mean ± SD), nor between all
aged women, 58 ± 23% and aged men, 49 ± 20%, were seen. However, the younger controls absorbed an average of 71 ± 19% of
the tracer, which was significantly different from the overall mean of 56 ± 25% for the elderly. Without knowing the
composition of the younger population (i.e. whether it was
made up primarily of menstruating women, who tend to be
marginally iron deficient), we cannot rule out an iron-sta-
tus effect, rather than an age effect as explaining the differences.

In Wales, Jacobs and Owen (1969) studied 36 non-anemic
individuals, 8 men and 28 women, ranging in age from 21 to
78 years. Whole-body counting after an oral dose of ^{59}Fe,
as either ferric citrate (nonheme iron) or radiolabeled rab-
bit hemoglobin (heme iron), both mixed into cream of chicken
soup, was used to calculate absorption of the isotopic iron.
The authors generated scatterplots of age versus fractional
absorption of isotope. As shown in Figure 1, there was an
almost linear decline in absorptive efficiency with increasing age with the inorganic iron test. With the heme iron
(data not shown), however, an equal rate of absorption was
seen across age. Transferrin saturation, as an index of
iron status was measured, and did not differ across age.
This study also suggests that intestinal capacity to absorb
iron decreases with age.

Contradictory results were found in the Dutch study by
Marx (1979). This investigator studied a total of 85 individuals using a sophisticated physiological iron absorption
test. It involved simultaneous administration to fasting
experimental subjects of 5 uCi of ^{59}Fe with a carrier iron
salt and 10 mg of ascorbic acid as a reducing agent, and
^{51}Cr as a non-absorbable fecal marker. Subjects were followed post-dosing by whole-body counting of the distinct
radiation energies of the isotopes in their bodies. Relating

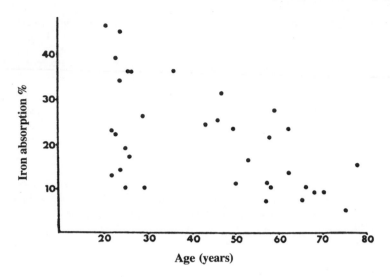

Fig. 1. Scattergram of non-heme (inorganic) iron absorption efficiency versus age in Welsh subjects. After Jacobs and Owen (1969). Reproduced with permission.

body content of radioiron and radiochromium at 1-h and 24-h postdose, allowed a calculation of both total intestinal uptake and mucosal transfer to the body's iron pool of the tracer dose of ^{59}Fe.

In the population sample of Marx (1979), there were 40 healthy active elderly persons, aged 65 to 83 y, 24 males and 16 females, with normal hematological status, and 25 young controls, aged 22 to 49 y, 15 males and 10 females, also with normal hematological status. Also included were 20 subjects with confirmed iron deficiency (and hence an increased affinity for iron), 14 below the age of 60 and six over 65 years of age. For the healthy subjects, comparative analyses were made by gender-group. The distribution of the rates of mucosal iron uptake, mucosal transfer, and net iron retention were found to be equivalent for non-anemic young and old, and were appropriately lower than those of the pooled group of young adults with iron deficiency. The interaction of the capacity to up-regulate iron absorption in the face of increased iron need in the elderly was also demonstrated by Marx (1979) in the finding of equivalently increased iron uptake, transfer and retention in younger and older subjects with iron depletion. Marx (1979), concludes that -- when iron status is carefully controlled for -- the absorptive capacity for iron is the same in both young and elderly.

Speculations

We can speculate that on *a group basis*, avidity of intestine iron uptake, both for diet and for isolated tracer doses would be lower in elderly than in the young. A possible explanation for this phenomenon would be, in the case of women, the habitual iron stores in a menstruating population. In males, a lower red cell turnover, due to a lesser active lean tissue mass and consequently lower oxygen transport demand in the elderly, would similarly explain any differences encountered.

Recommendations for Future Research

Indeed, high ascorbic acid intakes could induce an absorption of non-heme iron in excess of the needs of the aged individual. A survey relating supplementation practices with ascorbic acid, and body iron reserves would be useful to resolve this question. Appropriate down-regulation of iron absorption is suggested by the combined data on iron absorption in elderly presented above; what is not extensively documented is whether the *up*-regulation of intestinal iron uptake for repletion of an iron-depleted state is the same for older and younger adults. A comparative study in blood-loss anemia and iron absorption across ages would contribute additional important insights. Finally, as Jacob and Owen (1969) is the only study with *heme*-iron, absorption reported in the elderly, some extention of the observations on the handling of this form of iron in healthy ages subjects would be welcome.

ZINC ABSORPTION IN THE AGED

Biology of Zinc

Zinc participates in human physiology as a component of zinc metalloenzymes such as alkaline phosphatase, carbonic anhydrase, superoxide dismutase, etc. Zinc is vital to the biochemical processes of cell growth and cell division. It

is also important for the stabilization of membranes, in the
immune process, and in the conformation of polyribosomes
during intracellular protein synthesis. Zinc participates
in the physiological processes of growth, sexual maturation,
fertility, host-defense, sensory perception and bone development (Solomons, 1988). Its deficiency in man leads to
growth retardation and delayed maturation in children and to
hair loss, skin lesions, immune deficiencies, disturbances
of mood, nightblindness, impaired taste acuity and delayed
wound healing at any age (Solomons, 1988).

The average adult body contains from 2 to 3 g of zinc.
Of this zinc, that found in skin and bone is not available
for nutritional roles; the liver is probably the major depot
for metabolically-available zinc in the human body. Zinc is
transported in the circulation loosely bound to serum albumin.

Pertinent Aspects of Zinc Absorption

Zinc is absorbed along the whole extent of the small intestine. The divalent form of zinc, Zn(II), is highly stable, and is presumably absorbed in this form. At the intestinal surface membrane, both diffusion and a saturable
(carrier-mediated process) is involved in zinc uptake
(Cousins, 1987). The carrier-mediated process becomes important when dietary quantities of zinc are low. The control of zinc's release from the intestinal cell is exercised, in part, by the intracellular levels of the divalent
cation-binding protein, *thionein*. This protein traps excess
zinc, not required by the body's metabolism, and allows the
zinc to pass back into the intestine with the normal turnover of the enteral epithelial cell. For that zinc which
does pass into the bloodstream, an energy-dependent process
is required.

Various intraluminal factors are felt to influence the
biological availability of zinc. An *endogeneous* "zinc-binding ligand" (ZBL), of pancreatic origin, was postulated as
essential for the absorption of this metal (Evans, 1976).
A number of compounds have been posited as the chemical
mediator, but no conclusive identification has been made.
Food constituents such as dietary fiber, calcium, iron and
ethanol tend to reduce zinc uptake. Ascorbic acid has no
influence. Certain red wines may actually facilitate zinc's

absorbability (MacDonald and Margen, 1980).

The major route for excretion of endogenous zinc is also via the gastrointestinal tract. Zinc re-enters the fecal stream in the bile and in intestinal secretion, but princi- pally in pancreatic juice. Some of this re-excreted zinc is later reabsorbed; the remainder is lost in the stools. (Anonymous, 1981).

Changes in Zinc Absorption with Age

Studies of aging and zinc absorption in experimental animals has largely focused on the peri-natal period up to weaning (Solomons and Cousins, 1984). Methfessel and Spencer (1970), using a ^{65}Zn tracer and an aging rat model, reported a reduction in zinc uptake with aging in this laboratory rodent. In 1976, with respect to the situation in humans, Spencer et al. (1976) commented in a 1976 review: *"As both aging and various diseases may affect zinc status, the de- lineation of the effect of age per se and of various di- sease states becomes important.... As hormonal changes occur with aging, research on the effect of certain hormones on zinc metabolism may also contribute to the understanding of the changes in plasma levels of zinc in some physiol- ogical states, such as aging..."* Several *in vivo* studies published since that time have begun to address the issue of changes in zinc absorption with aging. In fact, zinc is re- presented by the greatest variety and abundance of human re- search in the elderly, including: 1) metabolic balance stud- ies, without and with isotopic tracers of zinc; 2) radio- isotope-based whole-body retention studies; and 3) plasma zinc uptake (zinc tolerance test) studies.

Several metabolic balance studies provide information on apparent absorption of zinc in elderly subjects. Three are from Berkely, California and involve the same six elderly men, aged 65 to 74 years, reported earlier in the context of iron (Turnlund et al., 1981; 1982a; 1988); the other emanates from the Departments of Human Metabolism and Chemical Pathology of the Medical Faculty of the University of Southampton, England (Bunker et al., 1982; 1984a). The latter studies involved 24 apparently healthy elderly subjects, aged 70 to 85 years. In one report, 10 subjects -- 5 men and 5 women -- were included (Bunker et al., 1982); in a second report, 14 additional subjects were added (Bunker

TABLE 2. Apparent Absorption of Zinc in Six Healthy
Elderly Subjects in the Berkeley Study

Metabolic Period	Mean Dietary Intake (mg/day)	Mean Fecal Excretion (mg/day)	Difference of Means (mg/day)
1	15.4 ± 0.3	14.1 ± 0.4	+ 1.3
2	15.5 ± 0.3	14.6 ± 0.5	+ 0.9

Modified after Turnlund et al., (1981)

et al., 1984a), for a total of 11 males and 13 females.
They ate self-selected diets. Collections of a duplicate
of the daily diet and of all feces excreted were made under
careful supervision in the homes over 5-day periods. Apparent absorption of zinc was similar for both reports. The
result from the larger series revealed a mean daily intake
of zinc of 8.9 ± 2.5 ug/day (range: 3.0 to 13.6 ug/day).
Fecal excretion averaged 8.5 ± 2.5 ug/day (range: 2.6 to
13.4 ug/day). Net apparent absorption was 0.4 ± 1.2 ug/day,
ranging from -2.6 to +2.4 ug/day. As a percentage of ingested zinc, apparent absorption averaged 4.3 ± 14.1%,
with a range of -39 to +25%.

The metabolic studies from Berkeley were conducted in
the in-patient facility, with subjects receiving a semi-
purified diet based on egg albumin, fed for several months
(Turnlund et al., 1981; 1982a; 1983). When one looks at
the comparable data on *apparent absorption* strictly from the
intake minus fecal output standpoint in the Berkeley elders
(Table 2), one finds a net daily absorption of 1.3 and 0.9
mg, respectively, for the first and second metabolic periods.
Again, a wide distribution among subjects of net daily zinc
retention was observed, ranging for -1.0 to +1.8 mg.

Turnlund and colleagues (1982a), in the same metabolic
experiments, examined the absorption of zinc using an
extrinsic isotopic marker (^{70}Zn) during the respective
balance periods. Fecal analysis was performed by thermal

ionization mass spectrometry. In elderly subjects, fractional absorption of the isotope was 17.3 ± 2.7% (± SEM)
combining all balance periods. This is equivalent to an
average of 2.6 mg of dietary zinc absorbed per day. The
individual values varied from -0.8 to +29.1%. In young
male subjects, aged 22 to 30 years, (number of subjects and
of balance periods not specified), consuming the identical
diet formula and stable zinc isotope under metabolic conditions, a significantly higher fractional absorption of ^{70}Zn
(31.4 ± 2.6%) was observed (p< 0.02). These young men,
therefore, absorbed about 4.7 mg of their dietary zinc. Thus,
although both groups maintained near zero overall zinc
balance, in the older men this was at the expense of a lower
uptake of dietary zinc into the body, presumably accompanied
by a lower re-excretion of endogenous zinc into the feces.

In all of the studies described so far, zinc was given
in a *dietary* context. Two studies have examined the efficiency of zinc absorption in a non-meal format, one using
radioisotopic zinc tracer, and the other an oral load of
zinc acetate   salts. The former study involved 75 normal
subjects studied at the National Institutes of Health over a
10-year period (Aamodt et al., 1983). This included   31
women and 44 men, aged 18 to 84 years, who received an oral
dose of carrier-free ^{65}Zn in the fasting state. Mean fractional absorption was found to be 65 ± 11%, with a range
from 40 to 86%. When the whole group was analyzed (Figure 2)
a clear decreasing trend was noted. The regression equation
was fractional absorption = 69.5 - *0.123 y* (where y = age in
years). This means that one loses 1.7% of one's initial
absorptive efficiency with each decade of life. When this
was disaggregated by sex (Figure 3), it was found that a
much more pronounced age effect was found in women. They
lost 3.2% of their initial absorptive efficiency per decade,
while the males only lost 1.9%.

In a study comparing young adult and elderly healthy
Texans, Bales et al. (1986) used the plasma appearance approach (or "zinc tolerance test"). In this report, subjects
ingested 25 mg of zinc as zinc acetate, in the fasting state.
Blood samples were collected at 60 min intervals over 4 h
following the dosing. Twelve young subjects in the age
bracket of 18 to 30, and 16 older subjects, all over 65 years
of age were compared. As shown in Figure 4, a statistically-
significant difference in the plasma zinc excursion at 2 and
3 h, and in the areas under the curve of plasma zinc uptake

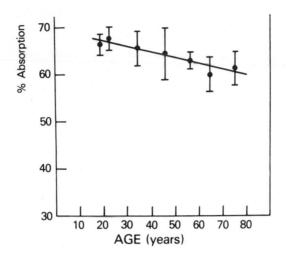

Fig. 2. Linear regression of zinc absorption with age. After Aamodt et al. (1983). Reproduced with permission.

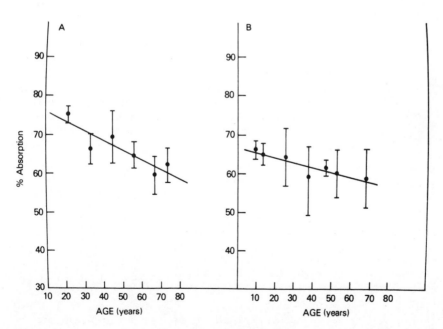

Fig. 3. Linear regressions for individual genders of zinc absorption versus age; A = women, B = men. After Aamodt et al. (1983). Reproduced with permission.

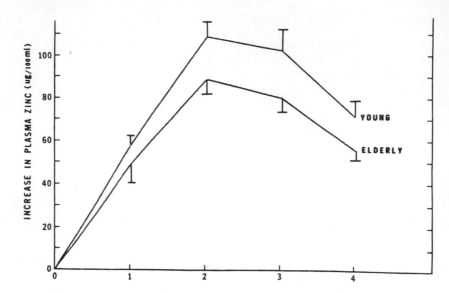

Fig. 4. Zinc tolerance curves in young and elderly Texans. After Bales et al. (1986). Reproduced with permission.

was observed, with the elderly having the lesser response. Similarly, the mean increase at the maximum post-dose concentration of plasma zinc was 188% above baseline in the young group, and 167% in the older group. It is most probable that these represent differences in intestinal absorption of zinc, but differences in tissue turnover or renal excretion related to age could also explain the differences observed in Figure 4.

Speculation

Since circulating levels of zinc decline in the elderly, and since daily intakes of zinc have been reported to be below RDA levels it has been *assumed* that the elderly were at risk of zinc deficiency. An alternative hypothesis, however, is that -- like iron -- zinc reserves accumulate over a lifetime. Thus, the diminished efficiency of zinc uptake documented in elderly (Aamodt et al., 1983; Bales et al., 1986), in physiological studies, could represent an *appropriate down-regulation* of zinc transport, analogous to that seen with iron.

Recommendations for Future Research

Should a more reliable indicator of zinc "reserves" become available (such as circulating of tissue levels of metallothionein), the hypothesis about the regulation of zinc absorption by the body's zinc reserves could (and should) be experimentally tested. The fractional absorption of zinc *from foods* needs to be explored experimentally in the elderly, as the only studies with diets extrinsically-labelled with isotopic zinc (Turnlund et al., 1983; 1988) used an artificial formula diet.

COPPER ABSORPTION IN THE AGED

Biology of Copper

Copper plays its physiological role as a component of various copper metalloenzymes. All enzymes of this class catalyze oxidation-reduction reactions involving molecular oxygen species; they include enzymes such as superoxide dismutase, lysyl oxidase and cytochrome oxidase (Solomons, 1988). Copper possibly has other metabolic roles, however, as not all of the physiological functions related to copper can be ascribed to specific, known cuproenzymes. These functions include: red cell and white cell formation; mitochondrial oxidative phosphorylation; skeletal mineralization; connective tissue formation; myelin formation; melanin pigment synthesis; catecholamine metabolism; thermal regulation; antioxidant protection; cholesterol metabolism; host immune defense; cardiac function, and glucose homeostasis (Solomons, 1988). Copper deficiency signs and symptoms in the state of human copper depletion include: hypochromic anemia; neutropenia; skin depigmentation; skeletal demineralization; subperiosteal hemorrhage; arterial aneurysms; hypotonia; and hypothermia. It is important to note that overt copper deficiency syndrome in an adult has never been produced based on a copper-restricted diet alone. Adult copper deficiency is seen either in the context of total parenteral (intravenous) alimentation with copper-poor solutions (Zidar et al., 1977) or with therapeutic or megadoses of oral zinc (Prasad et al., 1978; Patterson et al., 1985).

The body contains from 80 to 120 mg of copper (Mason, 1979), most of which is concentrated in the liver. Ceruloplasmin is a copper metalloprotein, and is the principal transport protein for copper in the circulation. Ceruloplasmin is an acute-phase protein, and infectious and inflammatory stress provokes a rise in circulating levels of ceruloplasmin. Relevant to the health of the elderly, it has been speculated by Goldstein et al. (1979) that circulating ceruplasmin exerts an anti-oxidant function by serving to eliminate superoxide radicals generated in the bloodstream.

Pertinent Aspects of Copper Absorption

Copper can be absorbed from the stomach and the upper intestine. In its usual form, bound to components of the diet, however, it is unlikely that copper (other than that dissolved in beverages) will be released into solution until the meal has reached the small intestine. Acidic pHs favor the dissociation of copper from food complexes. Copper absorption is a concentration-dependent, saturable process. The transfer step out of the intestinal cell is energy dependent (Crampton et al., 1965). Intracellular concentrations of the ion-binding protein, thionein, exerts a regulatory, blocking effect on the passage of copper out of the epithelium into the bloodstream. Braganza et al. (1981) have observed a relative *hyper*absorption of copper in individuals with pancreatic insufficiency, suggesting that pancreatic secretions may normally have a regulatory role in copper absorption.

Free histidine in the gut enhances the absorption of copper; copper is chelated by the amino acid, and taken up as a by-stander in the absorption of histidine. Cellulose interferes with the absorption of copper. Ascorbic acid has been shown to reduce copper bioavailability in a number of animal species (Solomons, 1985). Recently, in a primate model, Milne et al. (1981) showed that high doses of vitamin C interfere with copper absorption. Similarly, Finley and Cerklewski (1983) provide suggestive evidence that 1.5 g of ascorbic acid taken by human subjects will reduce copper bioavailability. One of the reported cases of human copper deficiency in a child was associated with chronic use of antacids. It was inferred from this observation that the alkalinization of the intragastrointestinal milieu could reduce the absorption of copper (Nishi et al., 1981).

The excretion of endogenous copper from the body is almost exclusively in the bile (Lewis et al., 1973). Biliary copper is poorly absorbable and is quantitatively lost in the stools. Thus, no effective enterohepatic circulation of copper exists. In cases of biliary compromise, copper accumulates in its hepatic stores (Shike et al., 1981).

Changes in Copper Absorption with Aging

The technical/methodological problems involved in assessing copper absorption studies has limited the number of copper absorption studies performed in humans of any age. The most widely used technique is the metabolic balance study, which gives *apparent* absorption values; given the important influence of biliary secretion of copper into the stools, the relationship of apparent absorption to true absorption of copper may be tenuous at best. More specific information about true absorption, per se, can be obtained in intestinal perfusion studies or using oral administration of radioisotopes, ^{67}Cu or ^{65}Cu. The invasive nature of these procedures, however, has limited their widespread use.

Two of the aforementioned metabolic balance studies provide information on apparent absorption of copper in elderly subjects: that from Southampton (Bunker et al., 1984a) and that from Berkeley (Turnlund et al., 1981). The details of both studies were provided in previous sections. For the 24 healthy elderly, collecting stools and diet duplicates at home over a 5-day period in Southampton, the average copper intake was 1.29 ± 0.56 mg/day (range: 0.65 to 3.05 mg/day) and the average fecal excretion was 1.32 ± 0.56 mg/day (range: 0.50 to 3.02 mg/day). The average apparent absorption was 0.04 ± 0.20 mg/day (range: -0.54 to +0.41 mg/day). Expressed as per cent absorption, this was -3.0 ± 16.7% (range: -35 to +38%), demonstrating marked interindividual variation. For the study involving 6 elderly men on the semi-synthetic egg-protein diet in Berkeley, the group mean results for copper intake and excretion are shown in Table 3 (Turnlund et al., 1981). Combining the two periods, the apparent absorption is a net of *zero*, but once again, there was considerable individual variability. A person who would have a consistent net daily loss of 0.1 mg of copper daily via the fecal route would deplete the 120 mg of adult stores of copper in just

TABLE 3. Apparent Absorption of Copper in Six Healthy
Elderly Subjects in the Berkeley Study

Metabolic Period	Mean Dietary Intake (mg/day)	Mean Fecal Excretion (mg/day)	Difference of Means (mg/day)
1	3.24 ± 0.14	3.18 ± 0.14	+ 0.06
2	3.28 ± 0.11	3.22 ± 0.06	+ 0.06

Modified after Turnlund et al. (1981)

over 3 years. Conversely, an individual with a constant net
intake of that amount would double his/her total-body burden
of copper over a similar span of time.

In the context of the Berkeley study (Turnlund et al.,
1982b), an attempt to approximate "true" fractional absorption of copper from the diet formula was made using a stable
isotope copper (^{65}Cu) tracer. Here, the same 5 elderly men
are compared with 6 young adult males. For the respective,
first and second metabolic periods in the elderly subjects,
the mean fractional absorption of isotopic copper tracer was
25.3 and 27.7%; for the respective periods in the young subjects, the copper absorption was 29.2 and 25.8%. These cor-
responded to net absorption of dietary copper of about 0.8
mg for the elderly men and 0.7 mg for the young controls.
Thus, across ages, no significant differences in copper absorption from this formula diets were seen.

An intriguing, but not fully interpretable, observation
on copper absorption and aging may be embodied in a comparison of three metabolic studies which focused on the *interaction* of zinc and copper, and on the competitive inhibition
of copper absorption by excessive amounts of dietary zinc
(Greger et al., 1978; Taper et al., 1980; Burke et al., 1980).
These studies do traverse the age-span. The study of Greger
et al. (1978) at Purdue was in adolescent girls receiving two
real-food diets -- one containing 11.3 to 11.6 mg of zinc and
the other 14.3 to 14.8 mg -- which provided 1.2 to 1.3 mg of
copper daily. Net copper retention was not influenced by the
higher zinc intake. Taper et al. (1980) at Virginia Poly-

technic Institute, studied adult women consuming 2.0 mg of
copper daily and, sequentially graded doses of 8, 16 and 24
mg of zinc; the increasing zinc consumption did not influence copper retention. Burks et al. (1980), also at VPI,
studied healthy elderly subjects. Their daily copper intake
was 2.3 mg, but zinc was varied at 7.8 or 23.3 mg. Apparent
absorption fell by 27% on the higher zinc intake in these
older subjects. This suggests that elderly may be more
sensitive to the antagonism of copper absorption by zinc
than younger persons.

Speculations

Unlike iron and zinc, copper has an efficient and responsive pathway for excretion from the body in the normally
intact biliary secretion process. This could be the reason
why copper, unlike the aforementioned trace metals, shows no
trend toward differential absorption with age.

Recommendations for Future Research

The fractional absorption of copper from foods needs to
be explored experimentally in the elderly, as the only studies with diets extrinsically-labelled with isotopic copper
(Turnlund et al., 1982b; 1988) used an artificial formula
diet. Ascorbic acid exerts a negative effect on copper uptake by the intestine. Given the prevalence of mega-dose
supplementation with vitamin C by the elderly, a study of
the interaction of copper status and the practice of high-
dose supplementation should be undertaken, analogous to the
study of Finley and Cerlewski (1983) in young adults.

SELENIUM ABSORPTION IN THE AGED

Biology of Selenium

The human adult body contains about 20 mg of selenium.
Selenium is a component of the selenoenzyme, glutathione
peroxidase (Levander, 1988), a key element in intracellular
antioxidant protection. This is the only selenoenzyme
confirmed in mammalian metabolism. The deficiency of selenium is characterized by myositis and cardiomyopathies,

hemolytic anemia, immune deficiencies. Recently, depigmentation of skin and macrocytosis have been described in selenium deficiency (Vinton et al., 1987).

Pertinent Aspects of Selenium Absorption

    There is only a relatively limited literature on absorp-
tive mechanism from experimental animal literature, and
only a few *in vivo* studies of selenium uptake in human subjects (Barbezat et al., 1984). The anatomic site for selenium absorption in humans has not been clearly defined. The
chemical form of the element is a major determinant of its
absorbability. Among the inorganic salts, *selenate* is more
bioavailable than *selenite* to humans (Thomson and Robinson,
1986). Neither form is as absorbable as organic compounds
such as *selenomethionine.* The latter is taken up by amino
acid transport mechanisms. Unlike the iron in heme, however,
the selenium remains associated with selenomethionine
throughout its transfer out of the enterocyte. The major
dietary form of selenium in both plant and animal foods is
selenoamino acids. No evidence for homeostatic regulation
of selenium uptake has been forthcoming (Barbezat et al.,
1984).

Changes in Selenium Absorption with Aging

    Studies on selenium absorption with an aging animal
model have not been reported. Two techniques have been
used to examine selenium absorption in humans: 1) with ^{75}Se
isotopes as salt or organic compounds (Thomson and Stewart,
1974; Heinrich et al., 1977); 2) with stable isotopic
tracers (Kasper et al., 1984; Janghorbani et al., 1984;
Solomons et al., 1986). There is also a literature on metabolic balance studied determining apparent absorption of
selenium (Greger et al., 1978b; Barbezat et al., 1984;
Thomson and Robinson, 1986). No data on aging effects have
been identified. One pathological condition, pancreatic
insufficiency (in the context of *juvenile* cystic fibrosis)
has been shown to reduce the efficiency of selenium absorption from cooked pork (Heinrich et al., 1977). Any loss of
efficiency in protein absorption with aging might influence
the availability of selenium; it would likely not be limiting.

Speculations

Ascorbic acid has been identified as enhancer of selenium absorption in experimental animals, but the question of
whether the reducing capacity of ascorbic acid might serve
to inhibit uptake of dietary selenium in humans by convert-
ing the intraintestinal species to a less soluble or less
absorbable form has been raised (Barbezat et al., 1984).
Among the nutrient-supplementation practices that has become
popular among the elderly is consumption of megadoses of
vitamin C. To the extent that ascorbic acid would exert an
inhibitory influence on selenium availability, problems in
the absorption of this nutrient might be seen in elderly who
take megadoses of the vitamin.

Recommendations for Future Research

Since no description of the aging effects on selenium
has been produced, the first priority would seem to be such
research. Both the *physiological* capacity for absorption
from a trace dose in aqueous solution and the efficiency of
uptake from the diet with an isotopically-labelled food
should be examined in normal healthy elderly. Interactions
with selenium uptake of medication commonly used by the
elderly should be studied as well.

CHROMIUM ABSORPTION IN THE AGED

Biology of Chromium

Chromium functions in mammalian nutrition in the potentiation of insulin action. It is essential to normal glucose and lipid metabolism (Anderson, 1988). Chromium is
normally transported in the circulation bound to transferrin.
The chemical form of the active chromium moiety that interacts with insulin biologically is not known with certainty;
it is believed to be a complex involving nicotinic acid and
amino acids. Clinical manifestations of human chromium deficiency have included fasting hyperglycemia, impaired glucose tolerance, glycosuria, elevated circulating insulin
levels, raised serum lipids, peripheral neuropathy, encephalopathy and inanition (Anderson, 1988).

Pertinent Aspects of Chromium Absorption

A summary of current knowledge of mammalian chromium
absorption has been provided by Mertz (1984). Chromium in
the form of trivalent chromic chloride salts is poorly
absorbed in humans, only to an extent of 0.5 to 0.7% of an
oral aqueous dose (Donaldson and Barreras, 1966; Doisy et
al., 1971). Chromium from organic forms in foods is considerably more bioavailable, as urinary excretion studies
reveal (Mertz, 1984). Absorption is most efficient in the
jejunum. Its cellular uptake and transport is by an energy-
independent, facilitated diffusion mechanism (Mertz, 1984).
The extent to which homeostatic regulation of chromium
absorption operates in deficiency or in overload is not
known. Competitive reactions of chromium with manganese,
iron and titanium have been demonstrated.

Changes in Chromium Absorption with Aging

Comparative studies of chromium absorption across the
age-span, from youth to old age, are not available. Bunker
et al. (1984b) in Southampton, England, have reported metabolic balance data and apparent absorption findings on
chromium. As with the previous Southampton studies (Bunker
et al., 1982; 1984a), these were again in home-living aged
consuming their accustomed diet. The total number included
22 healthy, elderly subjects. Only group data, but not individual values, were provided for apparent absorption.
Measured intakes ranged from 13.6 to 47.7 ug/day, with a
group mean of 24.5 ug/day. The fecal excretion ranged from
13.5 to 47.8 ug/day, with a mean of 23.9 ug/day. Thus, the
mean apparent absorption was +0.6 ug/day, but with a wide
variation from -23.5 to +12.7 ug/day. Two subjects were in
marked negative balance and three subjects were in marked
positive balance. The remaining 17 were close to equilibrium balance. A twenty-third elderly subject had mild
diabetes mellitus; she was in marked positive balance. It
is important to note that the average chromium intake for
these home-dwelling elders was only one-half of the lower
limit of the Safe and Adequate Daily Dietary Intake (NAS,
1980) for chromium. The Food and Nutrition Board established a 50 to 200 ug/day SADDI for this element. Since the
index is *apparent* absorption, the efficiency of true
chromium absorption cannot be assessed.

Both true diebetes mellitus and age-related impaired glucose intolerance are more common in the elderly. Doisy and co-workers (1971) showed that the plasma uptake of chromium from an oral dose was greater in insulin-dependent diabetics as compared to control subjects. Urinary excretion was also greater in the diabetics, and this response has been interpreted as a *compensatory* increased absorption to adapt to increased renal loss of chromium. This clinical observation argues, in fact, in favor of the existence of some form of homeostatic regulation of chromium absorption.

Speculation

If the technical capability to detect and discriminate subtle differences in intestinal chromium absorption was at hand, its application would reveal an inverse relationship between glucose tolerance and absorption of chromium from the diet in the elderly.

Recommendations for Future Research

The comparison of chromium absorption capacity across age should be undertaken. Efficiency of absorption of chromium *from the diet* is of highest interest. Urinary excretion of chromium must be suggested as the index of absorption; however, in the elderly, one must control for decreased renal clearance with an intravenous injection of radiochromium.

MANGANESE ABSORPTION IN THE AGED

Biology of Manganese

The human body contains an estimated 10 to 20 mg of manganese (Schroeder et al., 1966). Manganese is the metal component in two important mammalian metalloenzymes (Hurley, 1982). The first are glycosyl-transferases which are important for synthesis of glycoproteins in *mucus*; the second is the superoxide dismutase located inside the mitochondrion. In its soluble form, it also is a divalent cofactor in a number of reactions in carbohydrate and lipid metabolism. Only one, somewhat doubtful, case of human

manganese deficiency has been reported (Doisy et al., 1972).
Toxic intakes of manganese in humans occur in industrial
settings, and affected subjects show neurological changes
similar to those of Parkinsonism (Papavasiliou et al., 1982).

Pertinent Aspects of Manganese Absorption

The precise location of manganese absorption in the
gastrointestinal tract is not known, nor are the energetics
of intracellular events of manganese uptake well understood
(Hurley, 1982; Solomons, 1984). Iron, phytic acid and some
forms of dietary fiber may reduce its bioavailability.

Changes in Manganese Absorption with Aging

It is clear that manganese absorption evolves during
early post-natal life (Miller et al., 1975). Metabolic
balance studies have been conducted across the age-spectrum
from pre-adolescent girls (Engel et al., 1967), adolescent
girls (Greger et al., 1978), young adult women (McLeod and
Robinson, 1972), college-age men (Johnson et al., 1982) and
middle-aged men (Spencer et al., 1979). No studies in the
elderly are reported. Slightly positive balance was seen in
the first of the studies, and a slightly negative balance in
the last two. Either a gender, or a gender X age effect is
suggested. Since manganese excretion is also via the fecal
stream, the extent to which these metabolic balance studies
are reflecting *absorption* or *re-excretion* changes cannot
be judged from *apparent* absorption data alone.

Speculations

The consumption of tea by the elderly might assure a
suffcient amount of oral manganese for the body's needs no
matter how inefficient be the absorption.

Recommendations for Future Research

Given the absence of a human deficiency state, in the
overall perspective of trace elements in relation to geron-
tological health, manganese has a relatively lower priority
than some of the other nutrients mentioned.

REFERENCES

Aamodt RL, Rumble WF, Henkin RI (1983). Zinc absorption in humans: Effects of age, sex and food. In Inglett GE (ed) "Nutritional Biology of Zinc," ASC Symposium Series 210. Washington, D.C., American Chemical Society, pp 61-82.

Anderson RA (1988). Selenium, chromium, and manganese. (B) Chromium. In Shills ME, Young VR (eds): "Modern Nutrition in Health and Disease," 7th Edition. Philadelphia, Lea & Febiger, pp 268-273.

Anonymous (1981). On the enteropancreatic circulation of endogenous zinc. Nutr Rev 39: 162-163.

Bales CW, Steinman LC, Freeland-Graves JH, Stone JM, Young RK (1986). The effect of age on plasma zinc uptake and taste acuity. Am J Clin Nutr 44: 664-669.

Barbezat GO, Casey CE, Reasbeck PG, Robinson MF, Thomson CD (1984). In Solomons NW, Rosenberg IH (eds): "Absorption and Malabsorption of Mineral Nutrients." New York: Alan R. Liss, pp 231-258.

Bender AD (1968). Effect of age on intestinal absorption: Implications for drug absorption in the elderly. J Am Geriatr Soc 16: 1331-1339.

Bhanthumnavin K, Schuster MM (1977). Aging and gastrointes- tinal function. In Finch CE, Hayflick L (eds): "Handbook of the Biology of Aging." New York: Van Nostrand Reinhold, pp 709-723.

Bowman BB, Rosenberg IH (1983). Digestive function and aging. Hum Nutr Clin Nutr 37C: 75-89.

Braganza JM, Klass HJ, Bell M, Sturniolo G (1981). Evidence of altered copper metabolism in patients with chronic pancreatitis. Clin Sci 60: 303-310.

Bunker VW, Lawson MS, Delves HT, Clayton BE (1982). Meta- bolic balance studies for zinc and nitrogen in health elderly subjects. Hum Nutr Clin Nutr 36C: 213-221.

Bunker VW, Hinks LJ, Lawson MS, Clayton BE (1984a). Assess- ment of zinc and copper status of healthy elderly people using metabolic balance studies and measurement of leuco- cyte concentrations. Am J Clin Nutr 40: 1096-1102.

Bunker VW, Lawson VW, Delves HT, Clayton BE (1984b). The uptake and excretion of chromium by the elderly. Am J Clin Nutr 39: 797-802.

Burke DM, DeMicco TJ, Taper LJ, Ritchey SJ (1980). Copper and zinc utilization in elderly adults. J Gerontol 36: 558-563.

Cousins RJ (1987). Zinc metabolism - coordinate regulation as related to cellular function. In Taylor TG, Jenkins NK (eds) "Proceedings of the XIII International Congress of Nutrition" London, John Libbey, pp 500-504.

Crampton RF, Mathews DM, Poisner R (1965). Observations on the mechanism of copper by the small intestine. J Physiol (Lond) 178: 111-126.

Doisy EA (1972). Micronutrient controls on biosynthesis of clotting proteins and cholesterol. In Hemphill DD (ed): "Trace Substances in Environmental Health-VI." Columbia: University of Missouri Press, pp 193-199.

Doisy RJ, Streeten DHP, Souma JL, Kalafer ME, Rekant SL, Dalokos TG (1971). Metabolism of [51]chromium in human subjects. In Mertz W, Cornatzer WE (eds): "Newer Trace Elements in Nutrition." New York, Marcel Dekker, pp 155-168.

Donaldson RM Jr, Barreras RF (1966). Intestinal absorption of trace quantities of chromium. J Lab Clin Med 68: 484-493.

Duchateau J, Delepesse G, Vrijens R, Collet H (1981). Beneficial effects of oral zinc supplementation on the immune response of old people. Am J Med 70: 1001-1004.

Engel RW, Price NO, Miller RF (1967). Copper, manganese, cobalt and molybdenum balance in preadolescent girls. J Nutr 92: 197-204.

Evans GW (1976). Zinc absorption and transport. In Prasad AS (ed): "Trace Elements in Human Health and Disease." Vol 1 Zinc and Copper. New York, Academic Press, pp 1-188.

Finley EB, Cerklewski FL (1983). Influence of ascorbic acid supplementation on copper status in young adult men. Am J Clin Nutr 37: 553-556.

Frieman HD, Tauber SA, Tulsky EG (1963). Iron absorption in the healthy aged. Geriatrics 18: 716-721.

Geokas MC, Conteas CN, Majumdar AP (1985). The aging gastrointestinal tract, liver, and pancreas. Clin Geriatr Med 1: 177-205.

Goldstein I, Kaplan HB, Edelson HS, Weissman G (1979). A scavenger of superoxide of ion radicals. J Biol Chem 254: 4040-4045.

Greger JL, Zahie SC, Abernathy RP, Bennett OH, Huffman J (1978). Zinc, nitrogen, copper, iron, and manganese balance in adolescent females fed two levels of zinc. J Nutr 108: 1449-1456.

Greger JL, Marcus RE (1981).   Effect of dietary protein, phosphorus, and sulfur amino acids on selenium metabolism of adult males. Ann Nutr Metab 25: 97-108.

Harman D (1961). Prolongation of the normal lifespan and inhibition of spontaneous cancer by antioxidants. J. Gerontol 16: 247-254.

Heinrich HC, Gabbe EE, Bartels H, Oppitz KH, Bender-Gotze CH, Pfau AA (1977). Bioavailability of feed iron-(^{59}Fe), vitamin B_{12}-(^{60}Co) and protein-bound selenomethionine-(^{75}Se) in pancreatic exocrine insufficiency due to cystic fibrosis. Klin Woschenschr 55: 595-601.

Hurley L (1982). Clinical and experimental aspects of manganese in nutrition. In Prasad AS (ed): "Clinical, Biochemical, and Nutritional Aspects of Trace Elements," New York: Alan R. Liss, pp 369-378.

Jacobs AM, Owen GM (1969). The effect of age on iron absorption. J Gerontol 24: 95-96.

Janghorbani M, Kasper LJ, Young VR (1984). Dynamics of selenite metabolism in young men: studies with the stable isotope tracer method. Am J Clin Nutr 40: 108-218.

Johnson MA, Baier MJ, Greger JL (1982). Effect of dietary tin on zinc, copper, iron, manganese, and magnesium metabolism of adult males. Am J Clin Nutr 35: 1332-1338.

Kasper LJ, Young VR, Janghorbani M (1984). Short-term dietary selenium restriction in young adults: quantitative studies with the stable isotope ^{74}SeO$_3$(-2). Br J Nutr 52: 443-455.

Levander OA (1988). Selenium, chromium and manganese. (A) Selenium. In Shills ME, Young VR (eds): "Modern Nutrition in Health and Disease," 7th Edition. Philadelphia, Lea & Febiger, pp 263-267.

Lewis KO (1973). The nature of the copper complexed in the bile and their relationship to the absorption and excretion of copper in normal subjects and Wilson's disease. Gut 14: 221-232.

Lynch SR (1984). Iron: In Solomons NW, Rosenberg IH (eds): "Absorption and Malabsorption of Mineral Nutrients," New York: Alan R. Liss, pp 89-124.

MacDonald JT, Margen S (1980). Wine versus ethanol in human nutrition. IV. Zinc Balance. Am J Clin Nutr 33: 1096-1102.

Marx JJ (1979). Normal iron absorption and decreased red cell iron uptake in the aged. Blood 53: 204-211.

Mason KE (1979). A conspectus of research on copper metabolism and requirements of man. J Nutr 109: 1979-2066.

McLeod BE, Robinson MF (1972). Metabolic balance of manganese in women. Br J Nutr 27: 221-227.

Mertz W (1981). The essential trace elements. Science 18: 1332-1338.

Mertz W (1984). Chromium. In Solomons NW, Rosenberg IH (eds): "Absorption and Malabsorption of Trace Mineral Nutrients," New York, Alan R. Liss, pp 259-268.

Methfessell AH, Spencer H (1970). Effect of age and protein intake on ^{65}Zn excretion and tissue distribution in the rat. Radiol Res 43: 237.

Miller ST, Cotzias GC, Evert HA (1975). Control of tissue manganese: Initial absence and sudden emergence of excretion of the neonatal mouse. Am J Physiol 229: 1080-1084.

Milne DB, Omaje ST, Amos WH Jr (1981). Effect of ascorbic acid on copper and cholesterol in adult cynbomologus monkey fed a diet marginal in copper. Am J Clin Nutr 34: 2389-2393.

National Academy of Science (1980). "Recommended Dietary Allowances." Washington, D.C.: N.A.S.

Nishi Y, Kittaka E, Fukoda K, Hatono S, Usui T (1981). Copper deficiency associated with alkali therapy in a patient with renal tubular acidosis. J Pediat 98: 81-83.

Oski FA (1985). Iron deficiency - facts and fallacies. Pediat Clin N Am 32: 493-497.

Patterson WP, Winkelmann M, Perry MC (1985). Zinc-induced copper deficiency: Megamineral sideroblastic anemia. Ann Intern Med 103: 385-386.

Papavasiliou PS, Miller ST, Cotzias GC (1966). Role of liver in regulating redistribution and excretion of manganese. Am J Physiol 211: 211-216.

Prasad AS, Brewer GJ, Schoomaker EB, Rabbani P (1978). Hypocupremia induced by zinc therapy in adults. JAMA 240: 2166-2168.

Schroeder HA, Balassa JJ, Tipton IH (1966). Essential trace metals in man: Manganese. A study of homeostasis. J Chronic Dis 19: 545-571.

Shike M, Roulet M, Kurian R, Jeejeebhoy K (1981). Copper metabolism and requirements in total parenteral nutrition. Gastroenterology 81: 290-297.

Shock NW, Greulich RC, Andres R, Arenberg D, Costa PT Jr, Lakatta EG, Tobin JD (1984). "Normal Human Aging: The Baltimore Longitudinal Study of Aging." Washington, D.C.: U.S. Government Printing Office, NIH Publ. No. 84-2450.

Sirichakwal PP, Young VR, Janghorbani M (1985). Absorption and retention of selenium from intrinsically labeled egg and selenite as determined by stable isotope studies in humans. Am J Clin Nutr 41: 264-269.

Solomons NW (1984). Other trace minerals: Manganese, molybdenum, vanadium, nickel, silicon, and arsenic. In
Solomons NW, Rosenberg IH (eds): "Absorption and Malabsorption of Mineral Nutrients," New York: Alan R Liss, pp 269-
295.

Solomons NW (1985). Biochemical, metabolic oral clinical
role of copper in human nutrition. J Am Coll Nutr 4: 83-
105.

Solomons NW (1988). Zinc and copper. In Shills M, Young VR
(eds): "Modern Nutrition in Health and Disease," 7th Edition. Philadelphia: Lea and Febiger, pp 238-262.

Solomons NW, Cousins RJ (1984). Zinc. In Solomons NW,
Rosenberg IH (eds): "Absorption and Malabsorption of
Mineral Nutrients," New York: Alan R. Liss, pp 125-197.

Solomons NW, Rosenberg IH (1984). "Absorption and Malabsorption of Mineral Nutrients," New York: Alan R. Liss.

Solomons NW, Ruz M, Castillo-Duran C (1988). Putative
therapeutic uses of zinc. In Mills CF (ed): "Zinc in
Human Biology," Berlin, Apringer Verlag (in press).

Solomons NW, Torun B, Janghorbani M, Christensen MJ, Young
VR, Steinke FH (1986). Absorption of selenium from milk
protein and isolated soy protein formulas in preschool
children: Studies using stable isotope tracer, ^{74}Se. J
Pediat Gastr Nutr 5: 122-126.

Spencer H, Asmussen CR, Holtzman RB, Kramer L (1979). Metabolic balance of cadmium, copper, manganese, and zinc in
man. Am J Clin Nutr 32: 1867-1875.

Spencer H, Osis D, Kramer L, Norris C (1976). Intake, excretion and retention of zinc in man. In Prasad AS (ed):
"Trace Elements in Human Health and Disease," Vol 1 "Zinc
and Copper," New York: Academic Press, pp 345-361.

Steinheber FU (1985). Aging and the stomach. Clin Gastroenterol 14: 657-688.

Taper LJ, Hinners ML, Ritchey SJ (1980). Effects of zinc
intake on copper balance in adult females. Am J Clin Nutr
33: 1077-1082.

Thomas CD, Robinson MF (1986). Urinary and fecal excretions
and absorption of a large supplement of selenium: Superior-
ity of selenate over selenite. Am J Clin Nutr 44: 559-663.

Thomson AB, Keelan M (1986). The aging gut. Can J Physiol
Pharmacol 64: 30-38.

Trowell HP (1978). The development of the concept of dietary fiber in human nutrition. Am J Clin Nutr 31: S3-S11.

Turnlund JR, Costa F, Margen S (1981). Zinc and iron balance in elderly men. Am J Clin Nutr 34: 2641-2647.

Turnlund JR, Michel MC, Keyes Wr, King JC, Margen S (1982a). Use of enriched stable isotopes to determine zinc and iron absorption in elderly men. Am J Clin Nutr 35: 1033-1040.

Turnlund JR, Michel MC, Keyes Wr, Schutz Y, Margen S (1982b). Copper absorption in elderly men determined by using ^{65}Cu. Am J Clin Nutr 36: 587-591.

Turnlund JR, Durkin N, Margen S (1983). Zinc absorption in young and elderly men. Fed Proc 42: 850

Turnlund JR, Reager RD, Costa F (1988). Iron and copper absorption in young and elderly men. Nutr Res 8: 333-343.

Underwood EJ (1965). "Trace Elements in Human and Animal Nutrition," New York, Academic Press

Vinton NE, Dahlstrom KA, Strobel CT, Ament ME (1987). Macrocytosis and pseudo-albinism: Manifestations of selenium deficiency. J Pediat 111: 711-717.

Wagner PA, Jernigan JA, Bailey LB, Nickens C, Brazzi GA (1983). Zinc nutriture and cell-mediated immunity in the aged. Int J Vitam Nutr Res 53: 94-101.

Zidar BL, Shadduck RK, Ziegler Z, Winkelstein A (1977). Observations on the anemia and neutropenia of human copper deficiency. Am J Hematol 3: 177-185.

Mineral Homeostasis in the Elderly, pages 69–105
© *1989 Alan R. Liss, Inc.*

TRACE ELEMENTS IN THE ELDERLY

Ananda S. Prasad, M.D.

Department of Medicine, Division of
Hematology-Oncology and Wayne State
University School of Medicine, Harper-Grace
Hospitals, Detroit, Michigan, 48201 and the
United States Veterans Administration
Medical Center, Allen Park, Michigan 48201.

Abstract

    Amongst the trace elements, only iron, iodine,
zinc copper, chromium, selenium, manganese, cobalt,
and fluoride are considered to be essential for the
human health. In general, very little is known
concerning the metabolic effects of aging on trace
elements. It has been hypothesized that a marginal
deficiency of zinc and chromium may develop with
advancing age. Decreased dietary intake of zinc and a
decline in plasma zinc have been observed in elderly
subjects. In view of the known effects of zinc on
protein synthesis, gonadal functions in males and cell
mediated immunity, it is reasonable to speculate that
decreased testosterone level, problem with wound
healing, and anergy so commonly seen in elderly
subjects may be related to a marginal deficiency on
zinc. The adult onset diabetes may be related to a
deficiency of chromium inasmuch as chromium is
essential for glucose metabolism and a decline in
chromium content of tissues has been reported in the
elderly subjects. Whether or not a decreased intake
of copper plays a role in atherosclerosis and
increased aluminum intake is related to Alzheimer's
disease remains to be settled.

INTRODUCTION

    Several trace elements such as iron, copper, zinc,

chromium, selenium, manganese, cobalt, iodine, and
fluoride are known to be essential for human health,
but only a few have clinical relevance. Deficiency of
manganese in human subjects has not been established.
The only role of cobalt appears to be as related to
vitamin B^{12} molecule. Fluoride although important
for dental health, is not essential for life.

The essentiality of iron which is needed for heme
synthesis has been known for over one hundred years
and several reviews on this subject are available, as
such this topic will not be considered here. The role
of iodine in thyroid metabolism is also well known for
over a century and inasmuch as many books deal with
this subject, in this review iodine will not be
covered.

Deficiencies of zinc and copper in human subjects
have been recognized only during the past two decades
(Prasad et al., 1961; Prasad et al., 1963; Prasad
1978; Prasad, 1982). A great deal of progress has
been made in the understanding of their important
roles in biochemical functions. Clinical problems of
their deficiencies are being discovered with
increasing frequency in association with several
diseased states. Although clinical deficiencies of
chromium and selenium are not well established thus
far, their potential useful roles in clinical medicine
should be recognized.

In general, very little is known concerning the
changes in trace elements that may take place due to
aging. In the cases of zinc and chromium, it has been
hypothesized that with advancing age marginal
deficiency of zinc and chromium may develop. Recently
aluminum excess has been implicated in Alzheimer's
disease. In this review, the metabolic changes in
zinc, copper, and chromium due to aging will be
presented. The relationship of Alzheimer's disease
with aluminum excess will also be discussed.

Etiology of Zinc Deficiency

It is apparent that deficiency of zinc is
prevalent, accompanying inadequate protein intake such
as is seen in cases of protein-calorie malnutrition in
populations subsisting on low income and in geriatric
cases. Predominant use of cereal proteins by the

majority of the world population is an important predisposing factor for zinc deficiency. The availability of zinc in such diets is very poor because of high phosphate and phytate content.

Zinc deficiency in human subjects has been reported to occur in conditions where there is an increased requirement of zinc. These include infants and children during the rapid growth age period, and women who are pregnant and lactating. The recommended dietary allowance of zinc for infants, adolescents, and pregnant women are relatively high and it is unlikely to be met on an ordinary diet. Thus, physicians have to be aware of this possibility and take proper preventive measures.

Zinc deficiency has been reported to occur in patients with malabsorption syndrome. In such cases, deficiency of zinc is likely to occur in association with other deficiencies.

Hyperzincuria over an extended period may lead to zinc depletion. Conditions associated with hypercatabolic state such as surgery, burns, multiple injuries, major fractures, diabetes mellitus, protein deprivation, and starvation usually exhibit hyperzincuria (Prasad, 1978). Proteinuria and use of chelating agents such as penicillamine will also result in excessive zinc loss in the urine. Severe deficiency of zinc resulting from penicillamine therapy in a patient with Wilson's disease has been reported by Klingberg et. al. (1976). Hyperzincuria is likely to occur following chlorothiazide administration. Thus, hypertensive patients on long term therapy with chlorothiazide should be monitored for zinc deficiency. Glucagon is also known to cause hyperzincuria.

Patients with chronic liver disease, nephrotic syndrome and sickle cell disease are known to have hyperzincuria (Prasad, 1978; Prasad, 1982). It has recently been shown that several of the clinical manifestations of sickle cell disease and chronic liver disease are indeed due to zinc deficiency and zinc supplementation corrects these manifestations (Prasad, 1982).

Acrodermatitis enteropathica and sickle cell

disease, two genetic disorders, are known to be
associate with zinc deficiency (Barnes and Moynahan
1973; Prasad and Cossack, 1978; Warth et al., 1981;
Prasad et al., 1981). Severe zinc deficiency in
patients receiving long-term total parenteral
nutrition without zinc supplementation has been
reported by several investigators (Jeejeebhoy, 1982).
Symptoms are similar to those seen in acrodermatitis
enteropathica and include skin rashes, alopecia,
diarrhea, and depression. The onset of symptoms
usually 5 to 10 weeks after the start of total
parenteral nutrition is related to the severity of
zinc depletion in the patient.

Clinical Manifestations of Zinc Deficiency

Growth retardation, hypogonadism in males, poor
appetite, mental lethargy and skin changes were the
typical clinical features of chronically
zinc-deficient subjects from the Middle East as
reported by the author in the early sixties (Prasad
et al., 1961; Prasad et al., 1963; Prasad, 1982).
These features were corrected by zinc supplementation.

Recently, abnormal dark adaption in alcoholic
cirrhosis has been related to a deficiency of zinc
(Morrison et al., 1978). Zinc administration to
these patients corrected the abnormal dark adaption.
Similar clinical observations have been made in
zinc-deficient sickle cell anemia patients. It has
been proposed that the effect of zinc on the retina
may be mediated by an enzyme, retinene reductase,
which is known to be zinc-dependent.

In sickle cell disease, delayed onset of puberty
and hypogonadism in the males, characterized by
decreased facial, pubic and axillary hair, short
stature, low body weight, rough skin and poor appetite
have been noted and related to a secondary
zinc-deficient state (Prasad and Cossack, 1984; Prasad
et al., 1981; Warth et al., 1981). Many patients
with sickle cell disease develop chronic leg ulcers
which do not heal, and a beneficial effect of zinc
supplementation in such cases has been reported.

Some patients with celiac disease who failed to
respond to diet, steroids or nutritional supplements,
made remarkable recovery when zinc was administered.

They gained weight, and their d-xylose absorption test and steatorrhea improved following zinc therapy (Sandstead et. al., 1976; McClain et. al., 1980). Zinc supplementation in a few subjects with malabsorption syndrome (other than celiac disease) has produced beneficial results with respect to growth retardation, hypogonadism in males, mental lethargy, skin changes and loss of hair (McClain et al., 1980). One should, therefore, be aware of the occurrence of zinc deficiency as a possible complication of malabsorption syndrome.

The conclusion that zinc can promote the healing of cutaneous sores and wounds remained controversial for several years but most studies now provide evidence that zinc supplementation promotes wound healing in zinc deficient subjects and that zinc therapy in zinc-sufficient subjects is not effective for wound healing.

Abnormalities of taste have been related to a deficiency of zinc in many clinical conditions by some investigators (Henkin and Bradley, 1969; Henkin et al., 1976). Although a double-blind study failed to show the effectiveness of zinc in the treatment of hypogeusia in various diseases, another double-blind study indicated that zinc was effective in improving taste acuity in subjects with chronic uremia (Henkin et al., 1976; Mahajan et al., 1980). This discrepancy suggests that depletion of zinc may lead to decreased taste acuity, but not all cases of hypogeusia are due to zinc deficiency. The role of zinc in hypogeusia needs to be investigated further.

The dermatological manifestations of severe zinc deficiency include progressive bullous-pustular dermatitis of the extremities and the oral, anal, and genital areas, combined with paronychia and generalized alopecia such as seen in acrodermatitis enteropathica. Infection with Candida albicans is a frequent complication. These manifestations are seen in cases with severe deficiency of zinc.

Neuropsychiatric signs include irritability, emotional disorders, tremors, and occasional cerebellar ataxia. The patients generally have retarded growth and males exhibit hypogonadism. Zinc therapy has been shown to produce remarkable improvements and is considered to be a life-saving measure in these subjects.

A similar clinical picture has been reported in a patient receiving penicillamine therapy for Wilson's disease (Klingberg et al., 1976). Following total parenteral nutrition and excessive ingestion of alcohol, clinical manifestations of zinc deficiency resemble acrodermatitis enteropathica. Once a deficiency of zinc is recognized, zinc therapy becomes imperative in such cases.

According to Jameson (1980), zinc deficiency syndrome in pregnancy is characterized by increased maternal morbidity, abnormal taste sensations, prolonged gestation, inefficient labor, atonic bleeding, and increased risks to the fetus, especially post maturity. A possible correlation between maternal zinc deficiency and congenital malformations, especially of the central nervous system, has been postulated. A high incidence of congenital malformations has been observed in fetuses born of adult women suffering from acrodermatitis enteropathica.

In children recovering from severe malnutrition, limitation of lean tissue synthesis, with resultant obesity, and a propensity to infection are the major features of a mild zinc deficiency (Golden and Golden, 1981).

Biochemistry of Zinc

Studies by Vallee (1959) have shown that zinc is a constituent of several metalloenzymes. Keilin and Mann (1940) first showed that carbonic anhydrase was a zinc metalloenzyme. Later, it was shown that there is a single tightly bound zinc atom at the active site of this enzyme. During the next 20 years, only five additional metalloenzymes were identified. In the last 15 years, the total number has risen to 24. If related enzymes from different species are included, then more than 200 zinc dependent enzymes are now on record. Zinc enzymes are known to participate in many metabolic processes including carbohydrate, lipid, protein and nucleic acid synthesis or degradation. The metal is present in several dehydrogenases, aldolases, peptidases and phosphatases.

Zinc is required for both deoxyribonucleic acid
(DNA) and ribonucleic (RNA) synthesis (Slater et al.,
1971; Prasad and Oberleas, 1974; Dreosti and Hurley,
1975; Terhune and Sandstead, 1972; Fernandez-Madrid
et al., 1973). Many studies show that zinc
deficiency in animals impairs the incorporation of
labeled thymidine into DNA. This effect has been
detected within a few days after the zinc-deficiency
diet was begun. Prasad and Oberleas (1974) provided
evidence that decreased activity of deoxythymidine
kinase may be responsible for this early reduction in
DNA synthesis and may ultimately relate to growth
retardation. As early as six days after the animals
were placed on the dietary treatment, the activity of
deoxythymidine kinase was reduced in rapidly
regenerating connective tissue of zinc-deficient rats,
compared to pair-fed controls. These results have
recently been confirmed by other investigators
(Dreosti and Hurley, 1975).

Zinc may also play a role in the maintenance of
polynucleotide conformation. An abnormal polysome
profile in the liver of zinc-deficient rats and mice
has been observed. Acute administration of zinc
appeared to stimulate polysome formation both in vivo
and vitro. The data of Fernandez-Madrid et al.(1973)
who noted a decrease in the polyribosome content of
zinc-deficient connective tissue from rats and
concomitant increase in inactive monosome support this
finding.

Recent studies have shown that zinc plays a very
important role in cell differentiation and gene
expression (Miller et al., 1985). Earlier studies in
Euglena gracilis showed that zinc deficiency affected
growth, morphology, cell cycle and mitosis and it was
postulated that zinc played a role in gene expression
possibly through it's effects on zinc dependent
enzymes (Falchuk, 1988; Miller et al., 1985). It was
shown that in zinc deficient cells, the DNA content of
zinc deficient cells were twice normal, growth was
arrested and cells did not divide but remained
viable. The composition of mRNA was altered, and the
stability of the ribosomes with tRNA generated was
markedly decreased in zinc deficient cells (Falchuk,
1988). The zinc deficient cells contained only one
unusual type of RNA polymerase (x) as opposed to RNA

polymerase I, II, and III of zinc sufficient cells.
These studies suggest that zinc may have a selective
effect on gene expression. Both RNA polymerase, and
histones which bind to DNA and facilitate its
interaction with RNA polymerase are known to play
important roles in gene expression.

The ordered structure of chromatin is presumed to
be maintained by the binding of histones H_2A, H_2B,
H_3, and H_4 to DNA which results in a repeating
globular complex (a nucleosome) and by H_1 binding to
the intervening DNA segments between these complexes
(Falchuk, 1988). Significant changes in histones were
observed as a result of zinc deficiency in E. gracilis
and it was suggested that these alterations might
affect the binding of histones to DNA resulting in
either activation or repression of specific genes.

An essential part of gene expression and
regulation is the binding of a regulatory protein to
the recognition sequence of the appropriate gene.
Many such proteins have in their structures a domain
(or motif) which binds to DNA. Miller, McLachlan, and
Klug (1985) proposed that the xenopus transcription
factor III A contains small sequence units repeated in
tandem, and they proposed that each unit is folded
about a zinc atom to form separate structural
domains. Similar units have now been found in the
amino acid sequence of other transcription factors and
more generally, in nucleic acid binding proteins.
Thus, a second and apparently more commonly used
structure motif for DNA recognition has emerged,
conveniently called the "Zinc Finger". The role of
zinc in the DNA binding finger appears to be
structural.

The role of zinc in gonadal function was
investigated in rats (Lei et. al., 1976). The
increases in luteinizing hormone (LH),
follicle-stimulating hormone (FSH) and testosterone
were assayed following intravenous administration of
synthetic LH-releasing hormone (LH-RH) to zinc
deficient and restricted-fed control rats. Body
weight gain, zinc content of testes and their weight
were significantly lower in the zinc-deficient rats as
compared to the control. The serum LH and FSH
responses to LH-RH administration were higher in the
zinc-deficient rats, but serum testosterone response

was lower in comparison to the restricted-fed
controls. These data indicate a specific effect of
zinc on testes. Similar results have now been
reported in experimentally induced zinc-deficient
human subjects, sickle cell anemia patients, and
chronic uremics who are zinc deficienct (Prasad et
al., 1978; Mahajan et al., 1982). A decrease in
sperm count and serum testosterone level was related
to testicular failure due to zinc deficiency in these
human subjects. Supplementation with zinc resulted in
reversal of testicular failure in such cases.

Zinc has been used to isolate cell membrane and
neruotubules from rat brain, suggesting that it may
have a role on stabilization of plasma membranes
(Chvapil et al., 1972; Chvapil, 1976). Zinc prevents
induced histamine release from mast cells. This
effect of zinc may be due to action on the cell
membrane. Platelets are also affected by zinc ions.
Collagen-induced aggregation of dog platelets and
collagen or epinephrine-induced release of
^{14}C-serotonin, were significantly inhibited by
zinc. Supplementation of zinc to dogs effectively
decreased aggregability of platelets as well as the
magnitude of ^{14}C-serotonin release.

Several enzymes attached to the plasma membranes
control the structures and functions of the membranes
and the activities of these enzymes may be controlled
by zinc. Adenosinetriphosphatase (ATPase) and
phospolipase A_2 are inhibited by zinc which may
explain immobilization of energy-dependent activity of
plasma membrane or increased integrity of the
membrane structure.

In the erythrocyte, excessive intracellular
calcium causes shrinkage of membrane and hemoglobin
retention by erythrocyte membranes. Both of these
events may occur in sickled erythrocytes because of
sickling induced calcium accumulation. Zinc appears
to inhibit both of these events in sickled
erythrocytes (Brewer, 1980).

Many cell types are activated by calcium and
inhibited by zinc (Brewer, 1980). Examples include,
release of histamine by stimulated mast cells,
platelet aggregation and phagocytosis by neutrophils.
Zinc has been shown in inhibit the calcium ATPase of

the erythrocyte membrane. This enzyme serves as the calcium pump and is stimulated by calcium-activated calmodulin. The exact molecular mechanisms by which zinc inhibits calmodulin are not well understood.

Zinc and Immunity

Recent studies clearly indicate that zinc is required for lymphocyte transformation. Since Alford (1970) discussed the essentiality of zinc for phytohemaglutinin-induced transformation of human peripheral blood lymphocytes, several other laboratories have confirmed this observation. The effect of zinc appears to be that of a mitogen, and the kinetics of these influences most closely approximate the effects of antigen stimulation on lymphocyte culture. Currently available data suggest a direct stimulatory influence of zinc upon DNA metabolism, either by enzyme stimulation or by altering the binding of F^1 and F^3 histones to DNA so as to effect RNA synthesis. Direct cell surface effect of zinc, however, cannot be ruled out as a possibility. Zinc could be operating at several different levels in influencing lymphocyte monoclonal proliferation.

Assessment of the role of zinc in the development and functions of different lymphoid cell populations strongly indicate that this element has an effect predominantly on T lymphocytes (Good and Fernandes, 1979; Ruhl and Kirchner, 1978; Fraker et al., 1977). A monocyte factor may be required for the zinc-induced mitogenic response for T lymphocytes (Ruhl and Kirchner, 1978).

It has been known for many years that zinc deficiency in experimental animals results in atrophy of thymic and lymphoid tissue and lymphopenia. Fraker et al.(1975) first showed that severely and marginally zinc-deficient young adult A/Jax mice have involuted thymuses and reduced ability to form anitbodies to sheep red blood cells.

Iwata et al. (1979) have shown that one obvious hormonal effect upon thymocytes of zinc deficiency in mice and humans is reduction of thymic hormone levels which would clearly be another discrete local effect upon thymocyte maturation. Frost et al.(1977) have confirmed Fraker's observation of the reduction by zinc deficiency of T cell–mediated antibody production, but have also noted that the antibody production which occurs in deficient BALB/c mice is prolonged as compared to controls. This phenomenon may be explained by inhibition of T cell–suppressive function due to zinc deficiency.

Abnormalities of cellular immunity have also been observed in zinc deficient humans. An extreme example of the effects of zinc deficiency on the human immune system is acrodermatitis enteropathica, a genetic disorder of zinc malabsorption (Oleske et. al., 1979). This condition is characterized by muco-cutaneous lesions, diarrhea, failure to thrive, and frequent severe infections with fungi, viruses, and bacteria. Affected subjects have thymic atrophy, anergy, reduced lymphocyte proliferative response to mitogens, a selective decrease in T_4+ helper cells, and deficient thymic hormone activity. All of these changes are corrected by zinc supplementation (Chandra and Dayton, 1982). Less severe cellular immune defects have been observed in patients who become zinc deficient while receiving total parenteral nutrition. These abnormalities, which include lymphopenia, decreased ratios of T-helper and T-suppressor cells, decreased NK activity, and increased monocyte cytotoxicity, are readily corrected by zinc supplementation (Allen et. al., 1983).

In one study (Antoniou et. al., 1981), delayed hypersensitivity skin tests to mumps antigen were carried out in 25 apparently well nourished men who had a prior history of mumps infection and were receiving regular hemodialysis because of end stage renal disease. Nine patients were receiving zinc in the dialysis bath for treatment of hypogonadism. Only one patient in the zinc-treated group was anergic to mumps. In contrast, anergy to mumps and other antigens was observed in 11 of 16 untreated patients. Skin sensitivity test was restored to normal in three of four anergic patients treated with zinc.

Zinc deficiency occurs frequently in sickle cell anemia (SCA) subjects. Our studies have shown that several parameters of cellular immune function may be altered in SCA subjects and related to a deficiency of zinc. These include anergy to certain common antigens, which was reversible following zinc supplementation, decreased activity of natural killer (NK) cells, decreased production of interleukin (IL-2), and decreased T_4 to T_8 ratio. Inasmuch as we have observed similar immunological changes in human volunteers (non-SCA) in whom we restricted only zinc intake and produced a mild specific deficiency of zinc, we conclude that the above changes in SCA were due to zinc deficiency. Although it is well known that susceptibility to infections is a common problem in SCA subjects, the pattern of infections related to cell mediated immune dysfunction has not been well documented. Whether or not supplementation with zinc will atler the pattern of infection and decrease morbidity in SCA on a long-term basis remains to be determined.

A congenital deficiency of the purine enzyme nucleoside phosphorylase is associated with a severe T cell-immune deficiency. Our recent studies in experimental animals indicate that nucleoside phosphorylase may be zinc-dependent. Thus a decreased activity of nucleoside phosphorylase may additionally account for T cell dysfunction in zinc deficiency (Prasad and Rabbani, 1981). It is clear that zinc deficiency exerts a profound and apparently specific effect upon the thymus, thymocytes and cellular immune functions, which is reversible with zinc repletion.

The serum of animals or humans undergoing a bacterial infection contains a substance called leukocyte endogenous mediator (LEM) which causes a flux of serum zinc, amino acids and iron into the liver within a matter of hours following activation of phagocytic cells (Beisel, 1982). LEM is a low molecular weight protein produced by activated macrophages and granulocytes and may be identical to endogenous pyrogen (EP). The decline of plasma zinc is due to redistribution of zinc from the plasma pool to the liver. Hepatic uptake of zinc is accompanied by LEM-mediated synthesis by the liver of a acute-phase reactant proteins, such as ceruloplasmin, fibrinogen, a_1 antitrypsin and haptoglobin. Serum copper rises due to hepatic synthesis and release of ceruloplasmin. LEM also appear to mediate the release of neutrophils from the bone marrow. An increased number of blood neutrophils can be detected within eight hours after parenteral injection of LEM.

These alterations of zinc in acute stress may be significant, inasmuch as the reduced level of plasma zinc may increase the non-specific activity of local phagocytosis.

Recently, Briggs et al.(1982) showed that granulocytes from chronic uremics who were zinc deficient showed significantly impaired mobility, both chemotactic and chemokinetic, in comparison to those subject who were supplemented with zinc. Furthermore, a significant correlation between granulocyte chemotaxis and plasma and granulocyte zinc concentrations among all patients support a pathophysiologic relationship between the severity of impaired granulocytic chemotactic response and zinc deficiency in these patients. Abnormal granulocyte chemotaxis, corrected by zinc supplementation, has been observed by others in non-uremic patients with acrodermatitis enteropathica. It appears, therefore, that although the two neutrophil functions, phagocytosis and chemotaxis, are zinc dependent, their requirements for zinc are different.

Zinc may also intervene in non-enzymic, free-radical reactions. In particular, zinc protects against iron-catalyzed free-radical damage. The free-radical oxidation (auto-oxidation) of polyunsaturated lipids is most effectively induced by the interaction of inorganic iron, oxygen and various redox couples. Recent work suggests that this interaction underlies the pathological changes and clinical manifestations of iron toxicity. Zinc, ceruloplasmin, metalloenzymes (catalase, peroxidases and superoxide dismutase, a zinc and copper containing enzyme) and free-radical scavenging antioxidant vitamin E inhibit iron-catalyzed, free-radical oxidation.

Bettger and O'Dell (1981) observed that chicks fed a low-zinc diet developed severe skin lesions on the toes and foot pads as well as gross joint abnormalities. Supplementation of the zinc-deficient diet with vitamin E significantly reduced the severity of the skin and joint pathology, but had no effect on the decreased rate of growth in the zinc-deficient chicks. Their observations support the hypothesis that zinc plays an analogous biochemical role to that of vitamin E by stabilizing membrane structure and

thus reducing peroxidative damage to the cell.
Further studies in the red cell suggested that zinc
was not acting as an anti-oxidant, but as a stabilizer
of red cell membrane against damaging events that
occur following peroxidation.

Carbon tetrachloride-induced liver injury is
another animal model for studying free-radical injury
to tissues. Animals maintained on a high zinc regimen
are resistant to this type of biochemical injury,
suggesting that zinc may be protective against
free-radical injury. More recent studies have shown
that zinc also inhibits the analogous
metramidazole-dependent, free-radical sequence.

Some of the observed physiological effects of zinc
may be related to competition between zinc and several
cations such as cadium, lead, calcium and copper, both
in vitro and in vivo (Hill, 1976). Beneficial effects
of zinc on ameliorating toxicities of cadmium and
lead, accentuation of zinc deficiency by
administration of calcium and phytate, and production
of hypocupremia by excessive zinc intake, in human
and animal models, are some of the examples of
competition phenomena.

Zinc Status in the Elderly

Recent data from USA indicated that zinc intake
declines with advancing age (Sandstead et al.,
1982). Daily zinc intake may be as low as 7 to 8 mg,
whereas recommended dietary allowance for zinc in
adults is 15 mg a day. Abdulla et al.(1977) found the
zinc content of self-selected diet composites from 37
Swedish persons, all age 65 years, averaged 8.2 mg
daily. Other studies have also confirmed that in
general daily zinc intake of elderly subjects may be
lower than the younger adult population in Western
countries (Nationwide food consumption survey; DHEW,
1981). Several factors may account for this
observation. These include preference for cereal
proteins, decreased energy intake, and economic
restraint all of which have been noted in the elderly
subjects by some investigators (Sandstead et al.,
1982). It is well known that presence of phytates,
excess phosphate, and fiber in large quantities may
affect the bioavailability of zinc adversely from
cereal proteins (Prasad et al., 1961; Prasad et al.,

1963; Prasad, 1982; Prasad, 1978). Zinc intake is
known to correlate with energy intake, thus elderly
subjects who restrict calories, may become vulnerable
to marginal or moderate deficiency of zinc.

Suggestive clinical evidence of zinc deficiency in
the elderly subjects include decreased taste acuity,
poor appetite, mental lethargy, problems with wound
healing, higher prevalence of cell mediated immune
disorders, and hypogonadism in males which are known
to occur in elderly subjects.

Although a deficiency of zinc causing impaired
taste acuity in elderly subjects has been implicated,
the evidences to support this hypothesis are lacking.
A study of non-institutionalized and institutionalized
elderly persons (above the age of 69 years) revealed
no relationship between dietary zinc, hair zinc, and
taste detection of sodium chloride (Greger and
Sciscoe, 1977; Greger, 1977; Greger and Geissler,
1978).

The hypothesis that hypogeusia of the elderly may
be related to impaired zinc nutriture was tested
further by a double-blind zinc supplementation study
(Greger and Sciscoe, 1977; Greger, 1977; Greger and
Geissler, 1978). Forty-nine subjects (mean age 75
years) were supplemented with 15 mg of zinc or placebo
tablet daily for 95 days in addition to their daily
dietary zinc of approximately 10 mg. At the beginning
of the study, the taste detection thresholds tended to
be higher in the young adults and 8 per cent of the
subjects were unable to distinguish between deionized
water and 48 mM sodium chloride solution. At the end
of the study, no significant change in taste acuity
was observed in the experimental group. The
possibility that the zinc supplementation schedule did
not achieve adequate repletion of body store cannot be
ruled out and further studies are needed in the
future.

Wound Healing

The essentiality of zinc for collagen synthesis
and wound healing is now generally accepted (Pories
et al., 1976). This effect is primarily due to the
fact that zinc is essential for nucleic acid and
protein synthesis.

The occurrence of zinc responsive impaired wound healing is related to poor zinc nutriture in patients prior to hospitalization, increased losses of zinc that occur as a result of catabolism, and decreased availability of zinc for the diet and soft tissues store limiting the availability of zinc to the wound for healing purposes (Henzel et al., 1970; Cutchbertson et al., 1972; Lindeman et al., 1972; Fell et al., 1973). The severity of catabolism due to injury, influences the amount of zinc lost by excretion and the greater the injury and catabolism, the greater is the zinc excretion (Fell et al., 1973).

In one study, the serum zinc (mean $\pm$ SD) of 18 patients over the age of 60 yr preoperatively was 75 $\pm$ 15 ug/dl, whereas in 20 subjects under the age of 60 yr was 86 $\pm$ 8 ug/dl (p < .01) (Hallbook and Hedelin, 1977). It was noted that individuals with the largest wounds had the greatest fall in serum zinc post operatively, a finding probably related to a higher excretion of zinc.

In two double-blind zinc supplementation trials, improved healing of leg ulcers in elderly persons was observed (Haeger et al., 1974). In one study 29 patients (mean age 63.3 yr) with venous leg ulcers were treated with approximately 140 mg of zinc daily and compared to 28 patients (mean age 64 yr) who were given placebo. After 40 days of therapeutic trial, healing of the ulcers was significantly improved in the zinc supplemented group. In another double-blind study 13 patients (mean age 64 yr) received 600 mg zinc sulfate daily and 14 patients of comparable age received placebo (Hallbook and Lanner, 1972). This study showed that those patients who had serum zinc level less than 100 ug/dl, were benefitted by zinc supplementation so far as the healing of ulcer was concerned, whereas those who had greater than 110 ug/dl serum zinc level showed no beneficial effect of zinc. It is clear, therefore, that zinc supplementation must be given to zinc deficient patients who have problems with wound healing.

Immune Functions

Deterioration of T-cell immune function is known to be associated with aging (Duchateau et al., 1981;

Duchateau et al., 1981). The possibility that poor
zinc nutriture may contribute to this phenonmenon
exists. In one study 15 anergic institutionalized,
apparently healthy persons (mean age 81/yr) were given
100 mg zinc daily for 1 month, while 15 control
anergic subjects (mean age 79.6 yr) were given placebo
(Duchateau et al., 1981). The group receiving zinc
displayed an increased percentage of circulating
T-lympocytes, an increased frequency and magnitude of
delayed hypersensitivity skin reactions to purified
antigens, and a greater 1gG antibody response to
tetanus toxoid. No difference in phytohemagglutinin
or concanavilin - A stimulated in vitro lymphocyte
transformation was observed. Although the zinc
nutriture of the elderly subjects was not evaluated
and the relation of the changes observed to their
pre-study zinc nutriture is unclear, it seems evident
that certain aspects of cell mediated immune functions
were influenced beneficially in elderly subjects by
zinc supplementation.

The activity of lymphocyte ecto-5' nucleotidase
(5'-NT, a zinc dependent enzyme) has been observed to
decrease with advancing age (Boss et al., 1980). T
lymphocyte ecto 5'-NT activity begins to fall after
the age of 40 and subjects in the 61 to 75 age ranges
have only 38% of the activity present in younger age.
Thus, T lymphocyte ecto 5'-NT activity may be a
biochemical marker of immune system function in the
elderly. However, there is no evidence that the
activity of lymphocyte ecto-5'NT in any way determines
the immune system function.

An area of research which would be relevant to
zinc nutriture in the elderly is the apparent
influence of zinc status on the evolution of, or
resistance to cancer. Epidemiological studies in
humans suggest a relationship between zinc nutriture
and the occurrence of esophageal carcinoma (Anonymous,
1977; Lin et al., 1977; Kaplan and Tsuchitani, 1978;
Fong et al., 1978). In rats and mice a potentiation
of the carcinogenic effects of methyl nitrosamine on
the esophagus by zinc deficiency has been observed
(Fong et al., 1978). It is unknown if these findings
were related to the characterisitis esophageal mucosa
abnormailities as seen in zinc deficient rats or were
related to impaired immune functions as a result of
zinc deficiency in the elderly.

Burnett (1974) has suggested a role of zinc deficiency in senile dementia. He suggested that age-associated dementias such as senile dementia, Alzheimer's disease, Huntington's chorea, and the endemic neurological disease found in the chamorro people of Guam, might represent localized functional zinc deficiency. This hypothesis was based on the broader concept of "error catastrophes" as suggested by Orgel (1963) with the additional suggestion that lack of zinc would increase inefficiency and the occurrence of informational errors during replication of DNA or its activation for protein synthesis in somatic cells.

A recent study shows that intestinal absorption of zinc is decreased in older persons above the age of 65 year (Turnland et al., 1982). This may further indicate that subjects in older age group may be particularly vulnerable to zinc deficiency.

Although most studies have shown no association between plasma zinc and age, one study of 258 subjects, age 20 to 84 year, suggested that there is a declince in plasma zinc with age (Lindeman, 1971). Consistent with this were finding in 61 apparently healthy, ambulatory persons (mean age 71.7 year) who showed significantly lower plasma zinc levels than 71 control persons (mean age 31.4 year) (Sandstead et. al., 1982). In another study, the mean daily zinc intake of 36 women ages 66 to 96 year was 7.1 mg. The serum zinc level was decreased in this group (78 $\pm$ 2 ug/dl) and a negative correlation between age and serum zinc ($r = 0.519$, $p < .001$) was observed (Stiedemann and Harrel, 1980). In a few studies, the mean level of hair zinc in older persons was found to be lower than in young adults and adolescents (Sandstead et al., 1982). In one study, lower zinc levels in hair correlated with lower income (Wagner et al., 1981).

At present lower level of zinc in plasma and hair cannot be considered to be absolute evidences for zinc deficiency in elderly human subjects. Futher studies must be done in order to document zinc deficiency in elderly subjects. Also, careful zinc supplementation studies are required in order to document it's beneficial effects.

Recently we have recognized mild deficiency of zinc in elderly subjects between the ages of 65 to 85 years (Prasad, 1988). The diagnosis was based on their cellular zinc levels.

Inasmuch as plasma zinc is not regarded as a sensitive indicator of zinc deficiency if the zinc deficiency is mild, we assayed zinc in the granulocytes, lymphocytes, and platelets by recenlty established improved techniques in 23 randomly selected elderly subjects (ages 65 to 85 years) and were able to document for the first time mild levels of zinc deficiency in one-third of the cases studied. Mean values of the estimates of the nutrient intake for 24 hours of the 23 subjects were 1600 Kcal, 55.6 g protein, 64.75 fat, 17 g carbohydrate, and 7.8 mg zinc. Sixteen of the 23 subjects had zinc intake less than 10 mg per day, considerably less than RDA (15 mg/day).

The elderly subjects were further subdivided into two groups (mildly zinc deficient and zinc sufficient) based on their cellular zinc levels. A mild state of zinc deficiency was defined by a decreased level of zinc in any two cell types (lymphocytes < 48, granulocytes < 42, and platelets <1.7 ug/10^{10} cells). Normal levels of cellular zinc (mean $\pm$ SD) in our laboratory are as follows: lymphocytes 54.4 $\pm$ 6.6, granulocytes 49.8 $\pm$ 7.5, and platelets (2.2. $\pm$ 0.5 ug/10^{10} cells). By this criteria we observed that 8 elderly subjects out of 23 were mildly zinc deficient. Their zinc levels in plasma and erythrocytes were normal. In the zinc deficient group, 7 out of 8 showed anergy (less than 2 mm induration at 48 h to four antigens, PPD, tricophyton, mumps and candida), whereas 7 out of 15 subjects were anergic in the zinc sufficient group. The mean taste recognition threshholds for sodium chloride, sucrose, hydrochloric acid, and urea were higher in the zinc deficient group than those in the zinc replete group.

In the mildly zinc deficient elderly group, we observed not only a higher incidence of anergy and hypogeusia but also a decreased IL-2 activity of the T helper cells in comparison to the zinc sufficient elderly group (P <.001). The serum testosterone and dihydrotestosterone levels were significantly decreased in the elderly males when compared to male subjects between the ages of 20 to 40 years (p <.005). When the serum testosterone levels were compared between the mildly zinc deficient elderly subjects and zinc sufficient elderly subjects, it was significantly decreased (p< .005) in the zinc deficient group.

Our studies suggest that a mild deficiency of zinc may have possibly induced anergy, decreased IL-2 activity of the T helper cells, hypogeusia, and decreased serum testosterone levels in the elderly males. Our studies also demonstrate that measurement of zinc in cells such as lymphocytes, granulocytes, and platelets is useful in diagnosing mild deficiency of zinc in humans.

Whether or not aging per se affects zinc metabolism is not known at present. Clearly more studies are required in this field. A well controlled zinc supplementation study in the elderly must be carried out in the future in order to determine whether or not some or all of the zinc related clinical, biochemical, and immunological problems as discussed above are correctable. This may have a great impact on the nutritional management of the growing population of the elderly in this country and elsewhere.

According to Orgel (1963), random errors in protein synthesis occur at any age, but initially this phenomenon is probably of low frequency. The gradual accummulation of errors in various enzymes involved in nucleic acid and protein synthesis becomes amplified resulting in a decrease in cell functions or cell death with increasing age.

According to free-radical theory of aging as proposed by Harman, the cumulative delterious effect of free-radical reactions going on continuously throughout cells is a major contributor to aging. The observation that anti-oxidants extend the life span of some rodents provides support for the free-radical theory of aging (Harman, 1981).

In Burnet's model, the progressive weakening of thymus-dependent immune system responsbile for immunological surveillance was responsible for increased somatic mutations leading to cancer and autoimmune disease (Burnet, 1974). Walford (1980) also suggested that a somatic mutation in immunocytes leading to antigens modification may lead to increased incidence of auto immune disorders in aging population.

Inasmuch as zinc is know to be involved in DNA synthesis, in free-radical reactions and in cell mediated immunity, one may consider that an intracellular deficiency of zinc may play a role in the aging process.

COPPER

The presence of copper in plant and animal tissues was first recognized almost 150 years ago. Suggestive evidence of the dietary importance of copper in rats was first reported by McHargue in 1926 (McHargue, 1926) and in 1928 Hart el al.(1928) showed that copper, in addition to iron, was necessary for blood formation in rats.

The growth of young rats is retarded when they receive 3 ppm of copper in the diet. Young female guinea pigs on 0.5 to 0.7 ppm of copper grew well at first and their reproduction was equal to that of controls receiving 6 ppm of dietary copper daily. Eventually, however, they displayed a mild anemia, their hair coats became wiry and depigmented, and the growth of their offsprings began to slow down about the 12th day. Surviving animals on copper-deficient diet were markedly stunted by the 50th day of age.

Clinical Manifestations

Copper deficiency has been implicated in a syndrome affecting infants that is characterized by anemia, hypocupremia, and low serum iron and copper levels (Sturgeon and Brubaker, 1956). Combined iron and copper administration resulted in complete recovery. The hypocupremia was believed to result from an inability of the infants to obtain sufficient copper from a low-copper milk diet. During the past few years, copper deficiency has been reported in small premature infants, in malnourished infants alimented exclusively by the intravenous route, and in adults receiving total parenteral nutrition (Karpel and Peden, 1972; Vilter et al., 1974).

A full-term infant, or a premature of more than 1500 g at birth, does not become deficient on a low-copper diet without first experiencing prolonged and significant body losses of the element. These infants have normal concentrations of copper in the liver, which are adequate for many months after birth. On the other hand, the livers of small premature infants contain less copper, and are thus unable to meet the demands for rapid growth on a diet based on unmodified cow's milk containing low copper. With this simple exception, no instance of copper deficiency has been reported that has not resulted from prolonged diarrhea and poor dietary intake.

In Peru, prior to 1964, malnourished infants were routinely treated several months with modified cow's milk formula (Cordano et al., 1964). Because of relative lactose intolerance, the modified milk used to be diluted with sucrose and cottonseed oil. The water used to prepare the formula came from galvanized iron pluming but was deionized to control mineral imbalance. These factors undoubtedly accentuated the deficiency of copper. Cordano and Graham (1966) noted that infants on this formula, despite rapid growth and normal serum proteins (albumin and globulins), developed neutropenia and anemia. The abnormalities were corrected by copper supplementation.

Later in the course of copper deficiency, scurvy-like bone lesions (by x-ray) and occasional pathological fractures without any hemorrhage were observed. The existence of similar bone lesions, without anemia and neutropenia, in Menkes' syndrome (Menkes et al., 1962) which is believed to a congential defect in copper absorption, has not been explained. It is suggested that copper was available in utero for marrow development but not for calcified bone, central nervous system, or elastic tissue of the arterial vessels.

The peak incidence of copper deficiency in infants was under 1 year of age. This suggested that beyond that age, the infant or child was more likely to have consumed foods sufficiently rich in copper and the incidence of clinical deficiency was less detectable.

A clinical condition in infants, Menkes' kinky hair syndrome is an X-linked genetic disorder in which copper absorption from intestine is defective (Menkes et al., 1962). The disease is characterized by hypocupremia, a decreased level of copper in the liver and hair, progressive mental deterioration, hypothermia, defective keratinization of hair, metaphyseal lesions, and degenerative changes in the aortic elastin.

Deficiency of copper has now been reported to occur in adults who received total parenteral nutrition for several weeks without copper supplementation. Recently, copper deficiency characterized by hypochromic microcytic anemia and neutropenia was observed in adult patients with sickle cell disease who received 150 mg zinc daily in divided doses orally for nearly 2 years (Prasad et al., 1978). Zinc was primarily given for the healing of leg ulcer and control of pain crisis. Once recognized, the hematological changes were promptly corrected by administration of 1 mg copper orally daily.

Biochemistry

Cohen and Evlehjem (1934) showed that copper is essential for the synthesis of heme A, a component of cytcohrome oxidase, and thus copper was established as biochemically significant catalyst. An important cuprable protien was first isolated in 1938 although its function as an enzyme was not known until much later.

Since the isolation of hemocuprein, several copper-containing enzymes have been isolated and characterized (McCord and Fridovich, 1969; O'Dell, 1976). Some of these are cytochrome oxidase, superoxide dismutase, ceruloplasmin (ferroxidase), dopamine hydroxylase, and lysyl oxidase.

The role of copper in maturation of collagen and elastin is now well established. The major biochemical defect due to copper deficiency is a failure to form the normal cross-linking compounds in elastin and collagen. The formation of the crosslinking compounds of collagen and elastin is dependent on the oxidative deamination of the epsilon carbon of specific lysyl residues in polypeptide chains to form an aldehyde. Such reactions, involving molecular oxygen, are commonly catalzyed by amine oxidases. Recent evidences indicate that lysyl oxidase which catalyzes the conversion of peptidyllysine to the corresponding aldehyde residue is a copper metalloenzyme (O'Dell, 1976).

The daily turnover of copper approximates 0.6 - 1.6 mg and the daily requirement for adult man has been estimated to be 1.3 - 1.55 mg. (Wiliams, 1982). According to the recommendation of the National Academcy of Sciences, Food and Nutrition Board, the dietary intake of copper should exceed 2.0 mg/day. Recent dietary data, however, suggest that the daily copper requirement may not be met by many diets consumed in the USA (Williams, 1982; O'Dell, 1982).

Klevay (1973) first reported an elevation in serum cholesterol in rats fed marginal levels of copper with variable concentration of zinc. Excess zinc aggravates copper deficiency so that a high zinc to copper ratio increases the serum cholesterol level. Lei (1978) showed that copper deficiency elevates serum cholesterol but decreases the cholesterol level in the liver. Thus it appears that in nutritional copper deficiency cholesterol appears to be released from the liver more rapidly than normal but the metabolic basis of this hypercholesterolemia remains unknown. In cases of genetic copper deficiency, hypercholesterolemia is not observed.

Copper Status in the Elderly

Serum copper is known to increase with age (Lindeman, 1982). A similar increase in serum ceruloplasmin concentration also occurs. The mechanism by which serum copper increases with aging is not well understood at present. The existence of a reciprocal relationship between plasma zinc and copper in human and animal studies has been known for a long time, however, the exact biochemical mechanism for this phenomenon remains to be elucidated. Harman (1981) postulated that the increased copper, an excellent catalyst in the reaction of molecular oxygen with organic compounds, might enhance the rate of aging ("free radical theory of aging"). Increased production of free radicals might increase the rate of lipid peroxidation resulting in an acceleration of the process of atherosclerosis and arterio capillary fibrosis.

CHROMIUM

Etiology of Chromium Deficiency

Nutritional chromium deficiency has been suspected to occur in children in refugee camps in Jordan, and in malnourished children from Nigeria, and Turkey (Mertz, 1982). A few cases of chromium deficiency have been reported in subjects receiving long-term total parenteral nutrition (Jejeebhoy et al., 1977).

Multiparous women appear to have lower chromium store than nulliparae. Inasmuch as, in many countries nutritional intake of chromium may not be adequate, repeated pregnancies may further stress the nutritional chromium status of pregnant women. Whether or not deterioration of glucose tolerance in pregnancy is related to chromium deficiency, is not known.

Chromium deficiency should be suspected in diabetic cases where unexplained insulin resistance develops (Mertz, 1982). It has been reported that insulin (or stimuli that induce secretion of insulin) may mobilize chromium from unidentifiable tissue store. This leads to acute increases in plasma chromium levels and increased excretion of chromium in the urine. Thus, in case of hyperinsulinemia the chromium requirement is increased.

Clinical Manifestation of Chromium Deficiency

Impaired glucose tolerance is the major clinical manifestation of chromium deficiency. In a controlled study of 14 malnourished children in Turkey, the oral administration of 50 ug of chromium chloride, corresponding to approximately 50 ug of chromium, resulted in striking improvement of the impaired glucose tolerance in nine subjects (Jeejeebhoy et al., 1977).

It has been hypothesized that chromium deficiency may be a risk factor in atherosclerotic heart disease. Chromium supplementation in an uncontrolled fashion, has shown a decrease in serum cholesterol and a significant increase in HDL cholesterol level in adult subjects. Two additional epidemiological studies lend support to this hypothesis. One study carried out in Finland found a strong negative correlation between cardiovascular morbidity and mortality, and chromium levels. In another study low serum chromium correlated with increased incidence of coronary artery disease. Further studies are required to understand biochemical mechanism of the role of chromium in lipid metabolism and its significance in ischemic heart disease.

Diagnosis of Chromium Deficiency

Chromium determination in serum and other biological samples is not a readily available laboratory procedure. The results of such assays are not comparable from one laboratory to the other and assays are not well standardized.

No single test is currently available to assess the chromium status of individuals. Chromium status can be determined only retrospectively depending upon the clinical response of prolonged chromium supplementation in human subjects.

Dietary analysis of chromium in a given population may provide some knowledge with respect to adequacy of chromium nutrition. Normal intake for adults is 50 to 200 ug/day. A consistent intake below this range in any population increases the risk of chromium deficiency.

Analysis of hair, serum, liver, and urine for chromium have been utilized for assessment of chromium status. However, because of uncertainty of the techniques used for assay, it is not possible to relate the levels of chromium in these samples to body status of chromium.

Biochemistry of Chromium

Chromium is believed to be a co-factor for insulin. Chromium in the form of the naturally occurring dinicotinic acid glutathione complex (glucose tolerance factor), increased the effect of exogenous insulin on glucose metabolism epididymal adipose tissue in vitro. The effect of chromium is lacking in the absence of insulin.

Recent reports (Okande et al., 1981) suggest that chromium (III) may alleviate or regulate gene expression in mammals. Chromium was shown to bind preferentially to DNA in chromatin and cause an increase in the number of initation sites and thus enhances RNA synthesis.

Mertz et al. (1974) proposed that the biologically active form of chromium was comprised of chromium, nicotinic acid and possibly the amino acids glycine, cysteine, and glutamic acid. So far, however, conclusive evidence documenting the structure of biologically active form of chromium have not appeared.

Chromium Nutriture in the Elderly

Body store of chromium is known to decline with aging (Lindeman, 1982; Jeejeebhoy et al., 1977). This may be an expression of suboptimal chromium intake but a metabolic defect in chromium metabolism due to aging has not been ruled out. Further studies are required in order to relate chromium status in older subjects with abnormal oral glucose tolerance seen so frequently in older age onset diabetes.

A major stumbling block in studies of chromium metabolism in humans appears to be a lack of suitable technique for measurement of chromium in biological fluids. For instance, at present there is no agreement as to what are the normal levels of plasma chromium in humans. Clearly the first step is to establish reproducible methods of chromium assay before any progress could be made.

ALUMINUM

Aluminum has been implicated as a toxic factor in Alzheimer's disease. In this condition, there are several histopatholgic changes including neurofibrillary degeneration and senile plaques. The neurofibrillary degeneration is composed of pairs of 11 nm filaments arranged in helical array and differs from that found in the aluminum encephalopathy where it consists of 10 nm single filaments. However, other major histopathological findings of Alzheimer's disease, including neuritic plaques with amyloid cores, granulovascular degeneration and amyloid angiopathy cannot be explained by the known neurotoxic effects of aluminum. It is possible that in this disease the brain permeability is altered, allowing aluminum to accumulate. Interestingly, however, aluminum accummulates intranuclear and in approximately the same ratio as is found in the chronic toxic aluminum encephalopathy in the cats (Crapper McLachlan et al., 1983). A recent study of the effect of desferroxamine upon the clinical course of Alzheimer's disease indicated that prolonged treatment appeared to slow or arrest the course of this illness (Crapper McLachlan et al., 1983). Repeated measures of cognitive function employing the Wechsler Adult Intelligence score and Wechsler Memory Score, repeated measures of a signal detection task employing a backward masking paradigm, and repeated measures of electroencephalographic abnormality employing power spectral analysis were observed to be improved in this study. Obviously a larger clinical trial must be carried out in the future in order to assess the benefits of this mode of therapy.

Acknowledgements

Supported in part by grants from NIDDK, NIH, DK 31401, Bethesda, MD, the W.K. Kellogg Foundation, Battle Creek, MI, and the Veterans Administration Medical Research Service, Allen Park, MI.

Bibliography

Adbulla A, Jagerstad M, Norden A, Qrist I and Svensson S (1977). Dietary intake of electrocytes and trace elements in the elderly. Nutr Metab 21:41-4.

Alford RM (1970). Metal cation requirements for phytohemagglutinin-induced transformation of human peripheral blood leukocytes. J Immunol 104:698-703.

Anonymous (1977). Joint Iran-International Agency for Research on Cancer Study Group. Esophagel cancer studies in the Caspian Littoral of Iran. Results of population studies--a prodrome. J Nat Inst 59:1127-1138.

Allen JI, Perri RT, McClain CJ, Kay NE (1983). Alterations in human natural killers cell activity and monocyte cytotoxicity induced by zinc deficiency. J Lab Clin Med 102:577–589

Antoniou LD, Shalhoub RJ, Schechter GP (1981). The effect of zinc on cellular immunity in chronic uremia. Am J Clin Nutr 34:1912–1917.

Arakawa T, Tamura T, Igarashi Y, Suzuki H and Sandstead HH (1976). Zinc deficiency in two infants during parenteral alimentation for diarrhoea. Am J Clin Nutr 19:197–204

Bach JR (1981). The multifaceted zinc dependency of the immune system. Immunol Today 2:225–227.

Ballester OF and Prasad AS (1983). Anergy, zinc deficiency and decreased nucleoside phosphorylase activity in patients with sickle cell anemia. Ann Int Med 98:180–182.

Barnes PM and Moynahan EJ (1973). Zinc deficiency in acrodermatitis enteropathica. Multiple dietary intolerance treated with synthetic diet. Proc R Soc Med 66:327–329.

Beisel WR (1982). Single nutrients and immunity. Am J Clin Nutr 35:417–468.

Beisel WR (1982). The role of zinc in neutrophil function. In: Clinical Biochemical and Nutritional Aspects of Trace Elements. Prasas AS (ed) Alan R. Liss, New York, 203.210.

Bettger WJ and O'Dell BL (1981). A critical physiological role of zinc in the structure and function of biomembranes. Life Sci 28:1425–1438.

Boss GR, Thompson LF, Spiegelberg HL, Pichler WJ, Seegmiller JE (1980). Age dependency of lymphocyte Ecto-5' Nucleotidase activity. The J Of Immunology 152:679–682

Brewer GJ (1980). Calmodulin, zinc and calcium in cellular and membrane regulation: An interpretive review. Am J Hematol 8:231–248.

Briggs WA, Pederson MM, Mahajan SK, Sillix DH, Prasad AS, McDonald FD (1982). Lymphocyte and granulocyte function in zinc-treated and zinc-deficient hemodialysis patients. Kidney Internal 21:827–832.

Brummerstedt E, Basse A, Flagstad T, Anderson E (1977). Lethal trait A46 in cattle. Am J Pathol 87:725–738.

Burnet FM (1982) New Horizons in the role of zinc in cellular function. In: Clinical Applications of Recent Avances in Zinc Metabolism. Prasad AS, Dreosti IE, Hetzel BS (eds). Alan R. Liss, New York, 181–192.

Chandra RK, Dayton DH (1982). Trace element

regulation of immunity and infection. Nutr Res 2:721–733.

Chvapil M, Ryan J, Zukoski C (1972). The effect of zinc and other metals on the stability of lysosomes. Proc Soc Exp Biol Med 140:642–646.

Chvapil M (1976). Effect of zinc on cells and biomembranes. Med Clin North Am 70:799–812.

Cohen E, Elvehjem CA (1934). The relation of copper to the cytochrome and oxidase content of animal tissue. J Biol Chem 107:97–105

Cordano A, Baertl JM, Graham GG (1964). Copper deficiency in infancy. Pediatrics. 34:324–336

Cordano A, Graham GG (1966). Copper deficiency complicating severe chronic intestinal malabsorption. Pediatrics 38:596–604

Crapper McLachlan DR, Farnell B, Galin H, Karlik S. Eichhorn G, De Boni U (1983). In Biological Aspects of Metals and Metal Related Diseases. Sarkar B. Ed. Raven Press, New York 209–218.

Cuthbertson DP, Fell GS, Smith CM, Tilstone WJ (1972). Metabolism after injury. I. Effects of severity, nutrition and environmental temperature on protein, potassium, zinc, and creatinine. Br J Surg 59:925–931.

DHEW (1981). Health and nutrition examination survey No. 2. USPHA Division of Health Statistics, Hyattsville, MD.

Dreosti EI, Hurley LS (1975). Depressed thymidine kinase activity in zinc-deficiency rat embroys. Proc Soc Exp Biol Med 150:161–165.

Duchateau J, Delepesse G, Vereecke P (1981). Influence of oral zinc supplementation of the lymhocyte response to mitogens of normal subjects. Am J Clin Nutr 34:88–93.

Duchateau J. Delepesse G, Vrigens R, Collet H (1981). Beneficial effects or oral zinc supplemenation on the immune response of old people. Am J Med 70:1001–1004.

Falchuk KH (1988). Zinc deficiency and the E. gracilis chromatin. In: Prasad (ed.) Essential and Toxic Trace Elements in Human Health and Disease. New York, Alan R. Liss Inc., New York pp 75–91.

Fell GS, Fleck A, Cuthbertson DP, Queen K, Morrison C, Bessent RG, Hussain SL (1973). Urinary zinc levels as an indication of muscle catabolism. Lancet 1:280–282.

Fernandes G, West A, Good RA (1979). Nutrition,

immunity and cancer. A review. III. Effects of
diet on the diseases of aging. Clin Biol
9:91-106.

Fernandez-Madrid F, Prasad AS, Oberleas D (1973).
Effect of zinc deficiency on nucleic acids,
collagen and non-collagenous protein of the
connective tissue. J Lab Clin Med 82:951-961.

Fong YY, Sivak A, Newberne PM (1978). Zinc deficiency
and methybenzylnitrosamine-induced esohpageal
cancer in rats. J Nat Cancer Inst 61:145-150.

Fraker PJ, Haas S, Luecke RW (1977). Effect of zinc
deficiency on the immune response of the young
adult A/Jax mouse. J Nutr 107:1889-1895.

Frost P, Chen JC, Rabbani P, Smith J, Prasad AS
(1977). The effect of zinc deficiency on the
immune response. In: Zinc Metabolism. Current
aspects in health and disease. Brewer GJ, Prasad
AS (eds) Alan R. Liss, New York 143-150.

Golden MHN, Golden BE (1981). Effect of zinc
supplementation on the dietary intake, rate of
weight gain, and energy cost of tissue deposition
in children recovering from severe malnutrition.
Am J Clin Nutr 34:900-908.

Golden MHN, Jackson AA, Golden BE (1977). Effect of
zinc on thymus of recently malnourished children.
Lancet 2:1057-1059.

Good RA, Fernandes JA, Garofalo JA, Cunningham-Rundles
C,Iwata T, West A (1982). Zinc and immunity. In
Prasad, AS (ed.), Clinical, Biochemical and
Nutritional Aspects of Trace Elements, Alan R.
Liss, Inc., New York 198-202.

Good RA, Fernandes G (1979). Nutrition, immunity and
cancer - a review. Clin Bull 9:3-12.

Greger JL (1977). Dietary intake and nutritional
status in regard to zinc of institutionalized
aged. J Gerontol 32:549-553.

Greger JL, Geissler AH (1978). Effect of zinc
supplementation on taste acuity of the aged. Am J
Clin Nutr 31:633-637.

Greger JL, Sciscoe BS (1977). Zinc nutriture of
elderly participants in an urban feeding program.
J Am Diet Assoc 70:37-41.

Gross RL, Newberne PM (1980). Role of nutrition in
immunologic function. Physiol Rev. 60:188-302.

Haeger K, Lanner E, Magnusson PO (1974). Oral zinc
sulfate in the treatment of venous leg ulcer.
In: Clinical Applications of Zinc Metabolism.
Pories WJ, Strain WH, Hsu JM, Woosley RL (eds).

Charles C. Thomas, Springfield, IL 158–167.

Hallbook T, Hedelin H (1977). Zinc metabolism and surgical trauma. Br J Surg 64:271–273.

Hallbook T, Lanner E (1972). Serum-zinc and healing of venous leg ulcers. 2:780–782.

Hambidge KM, Hambidge C, Jacobs M, Baum JD (1972). Low levels of zinc in hair, anorexia, poor growth and hypogeusia in children. Pediatr Res 6:868–874.

Harman D (1981). The aging process. Proceedings of the National Academy of Sciences 78:7124–7128.

Hart EB, Steenbock, Waddel J, Elvehjem CA (1928). Iron in nutrition: copper as a supplement to iron for hemoglobin building in the rat. J Biol Chem 77:797–812.

Henkin RI, Bradley DR (1969). Regulation of taste acuity by thiols and metal ions. Proc Natl Acad Sci 62:30–37.

Henkin RI, Patten BM, Peter K, Bronzert DA (1975). A syndrome of acute zinc loss, cerebellar dysfunction, mental changes, anorexia and taste and smell dysfunction. Arch Neurol 32:745–751.

Henkin RI, Scheichter PJ, Friedewald WT, Demets Dl, Raff MA (1976). A double-blind study of the effects of zinc sulphate on taste and smell function. Am J Med Sci 272:285–299

Henkin RI, Smith FR (1972). Zinc and copper metabolism in acute viral hepatitis. Am J Med Sci 1972;264:401–409.

Henzel JH, Deweese MS, Lichti EL (1970). Zinc concentrations in healing wounds. Arch Surg 100:349–357.

Hill CH (1976). Mineral interrelationships. In: Trace Elements in Human Health and Disease. Prasad AS (ed) Vol. II Academic Press, New York 281–299.

Iwata T, Incefy G, Tanaka T, Fernandes G, Menediz-Botet CH, Pih K, Good RA (1979). Circulatory thymic hormone levels in zinc deficiency. Cell Immunol 47:100–105.

Jameson S (1980). Zinc and pregnancy. In: Zinc in the Envioronment, Part II: Heatlh Effects. J.O. Nriagu (ed). John Wiley, New York 183–197.

Jeejeebhoy KN (1982). Trace element requirements during total parental nutrition. In: Clinical, Biochemical and Nutritional Aspects of Trace Elements. Prasad AS (ed). New York, Alan R. Liss 469–476.

Jeejeebhoy KN, Chen RG, Marliss EB, Greenberg GR, and Bruce-Robertson A (1977). Chromium deficiency, glucose intolerance, and neuropathy reversed by chromium supplementation in a patient receiving long-term total parenteral nutrition. Am J Clin Nutr 30:531-538.

Karpel JT, Peden VH (1972). Copper deficiency in long-term parenteral nutrition. J Pediatr 80:32-36.

Keilin D, Mann J (1940). Carbonic anhydrase. Purification and nature of the enzyme. Biochem J 34:1163-1176.

Klevay LM (1973). Hypercholesterolemia in rats produced by an increase in the ratio of zinc to copper ingested. Am J Clin Nutr 26:1060-1068.

Klingberg WG, Prasad AS, Oberleas D (1976). Zinc deficiency following pencillamine therapy. In: Trace Elements in Human Health and Disease. Prasad AS (ed). Vol. I. Academic Press, New York 51-65.

Lei KY (1978). Oxidation, excretion and tissue distribution of (26-^{14}C-) Cholesterol in copper deficient rats. J Nutr 108:232-237.

Lei KY, Abbasi A, Prasad AS (1976). Function of the pituitary-gonadal axis in the zinc-deficient rats. Am J Physiol 230:1730-1732.

Lin HJ, Chan WE, Fong YY, Newbern PM (1977). Zinc levels in serum, hair, and tumours from patients with esophageal cancer. Nutr. Rep Int 15:635-644.

Lindeman RD (1982). Mineral metabolism in the aging and the aged. J Am Coll Nutr 1:49-73.

Lindeman RD, Bottomley RG, Conrelison RL Jr, Jacobs LA (1972). Influence on acute tissue injury on zinc metabolism in man. J Lab Clin Med 79:452-460.

Lindeman RD, Clark ML, Colmore JP (1971). Influence of age and sex on plasma and red-cell zinc concentrations. J Gerontol 26:358-363.

Mahajan SK, Abbasi AA, Prasad AS, Rabbani P, Briggs WA, McDonald FD (1982). Effect of oral zinc therapy on gonadal function in hemodialysis patients. Ann Int Med 97:357-361.

Mahajan SK, Prasad AS, Abbasi AA, Briggs WA, McDonald FD (1980). Improvement of uremic hypogeusia by zinc: a double-blind study. Am J Clin Nutr 33:1517-1521.

McClain C, Soutor C, Zierge L (1980). Zinc deficiency. A complication of Crohn's disease. Gastroenterology 78:272-279.

McCord JM, Fridovich I (1969). Superoxide dismutase. An enzyme function of erythrocuprein (hemocuprein). J Biol Cehm 244:6049-6055.

McHargue JS (1926). Further evidence that small quantities of copper, manganese and zinc are factors in the metabolism of animals. Am J Physiol 77:245-255.

Menkes JHM, Alter M, Steigleder GK, Weakley DR (1962). A sex linked recessive disorder with retardation of growth, peculiar hair and focal cerebral and cerebellar degeneration. Pediatrics 29:764-779.

Mertz W (1982). Clinical and public health significane of chromium. In: Clinical, Biochemical, and Nutritional Aspects of Trace Elements. Prasad AS (ed). Alan R. Liss, New York ,315-323.

Miller J, McLachlan AD, Klug A (1985). Repetitive zinc-binding domains in the protein transcription factor III from xenopus oocytes. Embo J 4:1609-1614.

Morrison SA, Russel RM, Carney EA, Oaks EV (1978). Zinc deficiency. A cause of abnormal dark adaptation in cirrhotics. Am J Clin Nutr 31:276-281.

Moynahan EJ (1975). Zinc deficiency and cellular immune deficiency in acrodermatitis enteropathica in man and zinc deficiency with thymic hypopasia in Fresian calves. A possible genetic link. Lancet 2:710.

Nationwide food consumption survey 1977-78. Preliminary report no. 2 (1980). Food and nutrient intakes of individuals in 1 days in the United States. USDA Science and Education Administration, Washington, DC.

O'Dell BL (1982). Biochemical basis of the clinical effects of copper deficiency. In Clinical, Biochemical, and Nutritional Aspects of Trace Elements. Prasad AS (ed). Alan R. Liss, New York 301-313.

Oleske JM, Westphal ML, Shore S, Gorden D, Bogden JD, Nahmias A (1979). Zinc therapy of depressed cellular immunity in acrodermatitis enteropathicas. Am J Dis Child 133:915-918.

Oleske JM, Westphal ML, Starr SS, et al (1979). Zinc therapy of depressed cellular immunity in acrodermatitis enteropathica. Am J Dis Child 133:915-198.

Orgel EL (1963). The maintenance of the accuracy of protein synthesis and its relevance to aging. Proceeding of the National Academy of Sciences 49:517–521.

Pories WJ, Mansour EG, Plecha FR, Lynn A, Strain WH (1976). Metabolic factors affecting zinc metabolism in the surgical patient. In: Trace Elements in Human Health and Disease. Prasad AS (ed). Vol. I. Academic Press, New York 115–141.

Prasad AS, Kaplan J, Abdallah J (1987). Zinc deficiency as a basis for immuno-deficiencies in sickle cell anermia (SCA). In Good RA and Lindenlaub E (eds.). The Nature, Cellular, and Biochemical Basis and Management of Immunodeficiencies. Symposium Medica Hoeschsl-21, Stuttgart - New York, FK Schatrauer Verlag 317–338.

Prasad AS (1978). Trace Elements and Iron in Human Metabolism. Plenum, New York p 251–346.

Prasad AS (1982). Clinical and biochemical spectrum of zinc deficiency in human subjects. In: Trace Elements in Human Health and Disease. Prasad AS (ed). Vol. I. Academic Press, New York 3–62.

Prasad AS (1982). Clinical disorders of zinc deficiency. In: Clinical Applications of Recent Advances in Zinc Metabolism. Alan R. Liss, New York 89–119.

Prasad AS, Abbasi AA, Rabbani P, Dumouchelle E (1981). Effect of zinc supplementation on serum testosterone level in adult male sickle cell anemia subjects. Am J Hematol 10:119–127.

Prasad AS, Brewer GJ, Schoomaker EB, Rabbani P (1978). Hypocupremia induced by large doses of zinc therapy in adults JAMA 240:2166.

Prasad AS, Cossack ZT (1984). Zinc supplementation and growth in sickle cell disease. Ann Int Med 100:367–371.

Prasad AS, Halsted JA, Nadimi M. Syndrome of iron deficiency anermia, hepatosplenomegaly, hypogonadism, dwarfism and geophagia. Am J Med 31:532–546

Prasad AS, Miale A, Farid Z, Schulert A, and Sandstead HH (1963). Zinc metabolism in patients with the syndrome of iron deficiency anemia, hepatosplenomegaly, dwarfism, and hypogonadism. J Lab Clin Med 61:537–549.

Prasad AS, Oberleas D (1974). Thymidine kinase activity and incorporation of thymidine into DNA in zinc-deficient tissue. J Lab Clin Med 83:634–639.

Prasad AS, Rabbani P (1981). Nucleoside phosphorylase in zinc deficiency. Trans Assn Am Phys 92:314–321

Prasad AS, Rabbani P, Abbasi A, Bowersox E, Fox MRS (1978). Experimental zinc deficiency in humans. Ann Intern Med 89:483–490.

Ruhl H and Kirchner H (1978). Monocyte-dependent stimulation of human T cells by zinc. Clin Exp Immunol 32:484–488.

Russel RM (1980). Vitamin A and zinc metabolism in alcoholism. Am J Clin Nutr 33:2741–2749.

Sandstead HH, Henriksen LK, Greger JL, Prasad AS, Good RA (1982). Zinc nutriture in the elderly in relation to taste acuity, immune response, and wound healing. Am J Clin Nutr 26:26:1056–1059.

Sandstead HH, Vo Khactu KP, Solomons N (1976). Conditioned zinc deficiencies. In: Trace Elements in Human Health and Disease. Prasad AS (ed). Vol. 1. Academic Press, New York 33–46.

Schloen LH, Fernandes G, Garofale JA, Good RA (1979). Nutrition, immunity and cancer. II. Zinc, immune function and cancer. Clin Bull 9:63–75.

Slater JP, Mildvan AS, Loeb LA (1971). Zinc in DNA polymerase. Biochem Biophy Res Commun 44:37–43.

Solomons NW (1981). Zinc nutrition and taste acuity in patients with cystic fibrosis. Nutr Res 1:13–24.

Stiedemann M, Harrel I (1980). Relation of immunocompetence to selected nutrients in elderly women. Nutr Rep Int 21:931–940.

Sturgeon P, Brubaker C (1956). Copper deficiency in infants. A syndrome characterized by hypocupremia, iron deficiency anemia and hypoproteinemia. AMA J Dis Child 92:254–265.

Tapazoglou E, Prasad AS, Hill G, Brewer GJ, Kaplan J (1985). Decreased natural killer cell activity in zinc deficient subjects with sickle cell disease. J Lab Clin Med 105:19–22.

Terhune MW, Sandstead HH (1972). Decreased RNA polymerase acitivity in mammalian zinc deficiency. Science 177:68–69.

Turnland JR, Michel MC, Keyes WR, King JC, Margen S (1982). Use of enriched stable isotope to determine zinc and iron absorption in elderly men. Am J Clin Nutr 35:1033–1040.

Valle BL (1959). Biochemistry, physiology and pathology of zinc. Physiol Rev 39:443–490.

Vilter RW, Bozian RC, Hess EV, Zellner DC, Petering HG
(1974). Manifestations of copper deficiency with
systemic sclerosis on intravenous
hyperalimentation. NEJM 291:188–191.

Wagner PA, Bailey LB, Krista ML, Jernigan JA, Robinson
JD, Cerda JJ (1981). Comparison of zinc and
folacin status in elderly women of differing
socio-economic background. Nutr Res 1:565–569.

Walford RL (1980). Immunology and aging. Am J of
Clinical Pathology 74:247–253.

Warth JA, Prasad AS, Zwas F, Frank RN (1981).
Abnormal dark adaption in sickle cell anemia. J
Lab Clin Med 98:189–194.

Williams DM (1982). Clinical significance of copper
deficiency and toxicity in the world population.
In Clinical, Biochemical, and Nutritional Aspects
of Trace Elements. Prasad AS (ed). Alan R. Liss,
New York 277–299.

Mineral Homeostasis in the Elderly, pages 107–111
© *1989 Alan R. Liss, Inc.*

Research Summary:

EFFECTS OF SIMULTANEOUS INGESTION OF CALCIUM AND MANGANESE IN HUMANS

Pao-Hwa Lin and Jeanne H. Freeland-Graves

Graduate Nutrition Division, University of Texas at Austin, Austin, Texas 78712

INTRODUCTION

The high incidence of osteoporosis in women has generated enthusiasm for the wide-spread use of calcium (Ca) supplements. Recently, a deficiency of manganese (Mn) has also been implicated in the etiology of this disease (Strause et al., 1986; Strause et al., 1987). Publicity of this association by the media may lead to increased use of manganese supplements by women as a preventative measure against osteoporosis.

Since several animal (Hawkins et al., 1955; Pond et al., 1978) and human (Spencer et al., 1979; Greger and Snedeker, 1980; McDermott and Kies, 1987; Friedman et al., 1987) studies have reported interactions between calcium and manganese, simultaneous consumption of these two minerals could possibly have competitive biological effects. The purpose of this study was to determine if concomitant ingestion of calcium and manganese in a supplement form would have an antagonistic influence on each other. An equivalent amount of calcium from milk was also tested since women may increase their use of this dairy product when concerned about their risk for osteoporosis.

METHODS

The effect of consumption of manganese and calcium on their respective absorptions were tested by a series of plasma tolerance (uptake) tests. Six healthy young adults were administered these tests. These studies were always separated by a minimum of 2 weeks to avoid any residual influence. At the beginning of each tolerance test, 5 ml samples of blood were collected from the antecubital vein of fasting subjects between 7 and 9 am. Then the subjects swallowed a gelatin capsule containing 40 mg manganese as manganese chloride and four more 5 ml samples of blood were drawn at 1, 2, 3, and 4 hours following the manganese load. Plasma was obtained via centrifugation in a clinical centrifuge at 3000 rpm and frozen at -70 ^{0}C until analysis for manganese. Standard precautions for avoiding trace mineral contamination were followed (Friedman et al., 1987).

The response from this initial manganese-only load served as the baseline manganese tolerance test for each subject. Further tests were conducted with the oral loads varying as either 800 mg calcium as calcium carbonate, 40 mg manganese plus 800 mg calcium, 545 ml of 2% milk, and 40 mg manganese plus 545 ml 2% milk. (A dose of 545 ml 2% milk was used since it contains 800 mg calcium.)

Plasma concentrations of manganese were determined by graphite furnace atomic absorption spectrophotometry (AAS) by methods previously described (Freeland-Graves et al., 1988). Total calcium levels were determined by flame AAS and ionized calcium by a calcium-sensitive electrode. Mineral concentrations in the blood are presented as the percentage increase in the sample from the initial fasting level. Changes in plasma concentrations were then tested for statistical significance using multivariate analysis of variance (Tabachnick and Fidell, 1983).

RESULTS

An oral dose of 40 mg manganese alone produced the typical rise in plasma manganese as shown in Table 1. With an oral load of manganese alone, the mean concentration of plasma manganese rose to its highest percentage increase over baseline values at the first hour postdose. The level of plasma manganese remained near a 100% increase for the second hour, then declined by approximately half at the third hour, followed by a further decline towards baseline at the fourth hour.

Administration of an oral load of calcium alone as 800 mg inorganic calcium in a gelatin capsule did not influence plasma manganese to any significant level. This lack of effect was expected. However, the concomitant ingestion of 40 mg inorganic manganese with the 800 mg inorganic calcium substantially blocked the uptake of manganese, as seen by a rise of less than 5% in the first hour and only 19% in the second hour.

When the equivalent amount of calcium (800 mg) was administered as 545 ml 2% fluid milk, plasma manganese was again unaffected. However, the addition of 40 mg manganese to the milk suppressed plasma concentrations of manganese to nearly the same extent, if not more so, than that seen with the simultaneous ingestion of calcium as the inorganic salt.

Table 1. Percentage increases of plasma manganese as compared to the fasting levels after different oral loads[1]

Oral loads	Hours postdose			
	1	2	3	4
40 mg Mn only	133[a]	97[a]	57[a]	23
800 mg Ca only	-30[b]	-16[b]	-21[b]	-15
40 mg Mn plus 800 mg Ca	4.6[b]	19[b]	-4.6[b]	-12
545 ml 2% milk only	-3.5[b]	-2.3[b]	-4.3[b]	-3.7
40 mg Mn plus 545 ml milk	-5.3[b]	-7.7[b]	-9.9[b]	11

[1]Values not sharing a common superscript within a column are significantly different ($p < 0.01$).

Concentrations of total plasma calcium rose slightly in response to a dose of both the inorganic and milk form of calcium. However, these slight changes were not statistically significant. The addition of manganese to the milk produced a smaller response in plasma calcium level compared to the inorganic salt. Plasma levels of ionized calcium did not change during any of these treatments.

DISCUSSION

The results of this study indicate that the simultaneous ingestion of calcium and manganese inhibited their respective absorptions in human subjects. This interaction occurred when manganese was in the form of an inorganic salt and calcium as either an inorganic salt or in 2% fluid milk. Plasma levels of manganese were affected more significantly than that of calcium, suggesting that calcium was the preferred ion.

Although the mechanism of the competitiveness between calcium and manganese is unclear, previous reports in animal studies (Hawkins et al., 1955; Pond et al., 1978) suggest that this antagonistic effect is valid. Furthermore, metabolic balance studies in humans have reported that manganese balance is affected by the level of dietary calcium (Spencer et al.,

1979; Greger and Snedeker, 1980; McDermott and Kies, 1987) and that serum levels of calcium are elevated in a manganese deficiency (Friedman et al., 1987).

These data suggest that taking supplements of these two minerals as single nutrients would have a greater effect on improving body status than if they were ingested as a combination. Although natural foods remain the ideal way to obtain nutrients, there are occasions when use of a nutritional supplement is appropriate. In this study, the best response in plasma uptake of manganese was seen when it was ingested as a single supplement.

The interacting effect of nutrients in combination nutritional supplements has been previously reported by Seligman et al. (1983). Iron in the form of a prenatal vitamin/mineral supplement was found to be less well utilized than that from a single iron supplement. The presence of calcium in the combination supplement was found to be partially responsible for this inteference.The results of the present experiment imply that calcium would also have a inhibitory influence on manganese if present in a multi-mineral supplement.

ACKNOWLEDGMENTS:

This work was supported in part by U.S. Department of Agriculture Competitive Research Grant 87-CRCR-1-2312 and University Research Institute, Biomedical Research Support Grant RR07-091-21.

REFERENCES

Freeland-Graves JH, Behmardi F, Bales CW, Dougherty V, Lin P-H, Crosby JB, Trickett PC (1988). Metabolic balance in young men consuming diets containing five levels of dietary manganese. J Nutr 118: 764-773.
Friedman BJ, Freeland-Graves JH, Bales CW, Behmardi R, Shorey-Kutschke R, Willis R, Crosby JB, Trickett PC, Houston SD (1987). Manganese balance and clinical observations in young men fed a manganese-deficient diet. J Nutr 117: 133-143.
Greger JL, Snedeker SM (1980). Effect of dietary protein and phosphorus levels on the utilization of zinc, copper, and manganese by adult males. J Nutr 110: 2243-2253.
Hawkins GE, Wise GH, Matrone G, Waugh RK (1955). Manganese in the nutrition of young dairy cattle fed different levels of calcium and phosphorus. J Dairy Sci 38: 536-547.

McDermott SD, Kies C (1987). Manganese usage in humans as affected by use of calcium supplements. In Kies C (ed): "Nutritional Bioavailability of Manganese," Washington, DC: American Chemical Society, pp 141-151.

Pond WG, Walker EF Jr, Kirtland D (1978). Effect of dietary calcium and phosphorus level from 40 to 100 Kg body weight gain and bone and soft tissue mineral concentrations. J Anim Sci 46: 686-691.

Seligman PA, Caskey JH, Frazier JL, Zucker RM, Podell R, Allen RH (1983). Measurements of iron absorption from prenatal multivitamin-mineral supplements. Obset Gynecol 61: 356-362.

Spencer H, Asmussen CR, Holtzman RB, Kramer L (1979). Metabolic balances of Cd, Cu, Mn, and Zn in man. Am J Clin Nutr 32: 1867-1875.

Strause LG, Hegenauer J, Saltman P, Cone R, Resnick D (1986). Effects of long-term dietary manganese and copper deficiency on rat skeleton. J Nutr 116: 135-141.

Strause L, Saltman P, Glowacki J (1987). The effect of deficiencies of manganese and copper on osteoinduction and on resorption of bone particles in rats. Calcif Tissue Int 41: 145-150.

Tabachnick BG, Fidell LS (1983). "Using Multivariate Statistics," New York: Harper and Row Publishers.

EFFECT OF AGING ON MINERAL METABOLISM AND REQUIREMENTS

Mineral Homeostasis in the Elderly, pages 115–126
© 1989 Alan R. Liss, Inc.

NUTRITIONAL CONSIDERATIONS IN BONE HEALTH AND AGING

Robert P. Heaney, M.D., F.A.C.P.

Creighton University, Omaha, Nebraska

THE OSTEOPOROTIC FRACTURE CONTEXT

The principal concern of bone health in the aging is structural. Can the skeleton remain strong enough to resist ordinary loads without fracturing? When bones collapse under normal loads, the diagnosis most often is "osteoporosis" - a term that means literally that the bones are porous.

Structures, whether bones, bridges, or buildings, are designed to carry a certain amount of weight and resist certain mechanical forces. They fail for three main reasons:

¤ they contain too little structural material;

¤ the materials used are intrinsically weak to begin with or they develop defects with use which render them weak;

¤ the materials, even though adequate in quantity and quality, are assembled poorly, or some of their connections are lost with use, so that the structure is not as strong as it appears.

All three reasons apply to the problem of osteoporosis, just as they do to failure in engineering structures. The first - a decrease in the quantity of bone - is the one that has given its name to the problem and has dominated the attention of osteoporosis investigators for the past fifty years.

The second reason - a defect in the quality of the bony material - occurs whenever repeated use weakens the bone through a process known to structures engineers as "fatigue damage." This problem has been much in the news in recent years, because it has been responsible for the failure of critical parts in airplanes and bridges. The same type of damage occurs in human bone: every time we load our skeletons, the bone bends. This deformation is typically on the order of about 1-2 parts in a thousand, still, after a few thousands of loading cycles, tiny cracks develop and the material gradually weakens (Carter DR, Caler WE, et al. 1981). Fatigue damage does not normally accumulate in bone - at least to the point of overt failure - because the process of bone remodeling detects the damage, removes the affected bone, and replaces it with fresh new bone. However, when remodeling fails for any reason, fatigue damage accumulates and the bone gets progressively weaker, irrespective of changes in mass.

The third cause of weakness, defective structural arrangement, also occurs in bone just as it does in engineering structures. It is a problem specifically of trabecular bone. Trabecular structures can be very strong, even when the bony material occupies only a small fraction of the total volume. But that strength depends upon the integrity of all the connections. For example, in normal bone, vertical trabeculae are braced by horizontal elements that keep the vertical ones from bending too much when loaded along their axis. Disconnect those horizontal beams, and the vertical ones become very flimsy. Exactly this process occurs in many persons with the vertebral crush fracture syndrome typical of osteoporosis (Aaron JE, Makins NB, et al. 1987; (Kleerekoper M, Feldkamp LA, et al. 1987). Other people, with the same amount of bone loss, but with those critical trabecular connections still intact, do not fracture.

The point of all this is that, while we once thought of osteoporosis simply as a decrease in the amount of bone, we have now come to recognize that the problem is more complex and that whether a woman develops an osteoporotic fracture depends not only upon the amount of bone she has, but upon the amount of fatigue damage which has accumulated in that bone, and on the structural integrity of the critical connections that give the structure much of its strength. As might be expected, all three of these factors interact (Fig. 1). A decrease in the amount of bone present in the skeleton allows the bone to bend more and in this way causes more fatigue damage. This of course only aggravates the fragility. So, too, flimsiness of the trabeculae certainly aggravates the problem of structural disconnection.

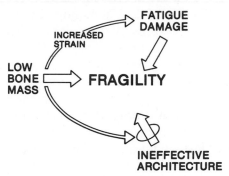

Fig. 1. Interaction of principal factors in bone fragility. All three directly weaken bone. Additionally, decreased mass leads to increased fatigue damage because, with constant loading, thin structures deform more than thick ones. (Copyright, 1988, Robert P. Heaney. Used with permission.)

The belated recognition that there are other contributing causes of fragility helps explain not only why some people with low bone mass develop fractures and others do not, but also why bone scanning for the early detection of osteoporosis is so often a waste of time and money. For bone scans measure only one of the reasons bones are fragile, the decrease in bone mass. They tell us nothing about fatigue damage or structural connectivity.

Bone mass is still an important part of the problem, for people with heavy, dense skeletons can tolerate more fatigue damage and structural disconnection than can those with fragile skeletons. Furthermore, bone mass is the only component of bone fragility that is easily measurable or that medical science knows much about. Hence, in the remainder of this chapter, I shall be forced to concentrate predominantly on factors that influence the amount of bone a person has. And more specifically, bone mass is the only fragility-related factor for which there are currently recognized nutritional interactions.

BONE MASS AND BONE LOSS

All persons lose bone with age. The process begins slowly, probably at about age 35-40, and occurs in both men and women. The loss initially is about 0.3-0.6% per year. But at menopause in women there is a very considerable acceleration of this loss. This rapid post-menopausal loss gradually slows until, by age 70-75, the woman is back to the old rate of about 0.3-0.6% per year. Three reasons for these losses are currently recognized: 1) physical inactivity, 2) loss of sex hormones, particularly, in women, estrogen at the time of menopause, and 3) inadequate intake of basic nutrients, mainly calcium.

Physical activity is just as important for bone health as it is for muscle strength. One of the best kept secrets of this field is the fact that there is a nearly constant ratio of bone to muscle in a woman's body. Women who have a subnormal amount of bone, in the condition we call osteoporosis, have an equally subnormal amount of muscle. This association underscores the importance of a life-long program of vigorous physical activity.

The second factor is the loss of gonadal hormones. This is an unusual occurrence in men, but occurs routinely in women at menopause. In both sexes, however, it results in bone loss. The precise mechanism remains obscure, but the phenomenon has been so well studied, and is so reproducible, that there can be no doubt about the fundamental facts: 1) a woman loses from 10 to 20 percent of the bone in critical portions of her skeleton in the 10 to 15 years following menopause; and 2) this component of age-related loss can be prevented by estrogen replacement therapy (ERT), essentially indefinitely - or at least until the ERT itself is stopped.

The third factor is nutritional deficiency, particularly calcium deficiency. The mineral component of bone substance is a complex salt made up mostly of calcium, phosphate, and carbonate. Phosphate is rarely limiting in human nutrition, but calcium often is. Calcium deficiency causes bone loss simply because the body treats bone as a seemingly limitless reservoir of calcium, upon which it can draw in order to support the level of calcium in the extracellular fluid. If our diets do not contain enough calcium, if we fail to absorb diet calcium efficiently, or if we lose excessive amounts of calcium through high obligatory excretory losses, then the calcium homeostatic system turns to the bones as its backup source of calcium. Parathyroid hormone activates the bone remodeling process and scavenges the calcium that is released as a byproduct of the destructive, first phase of bone remodeling.

There are other nutrients important for bone health in addition to calcium. These include trace elements such as manganese, zinc, and copper. More recently boron has been implicated as an important nutrient, helping the body conserve calcium and even reinforcing the calcium-conserving effect of the sex hormones (Nielsen FH, Hunt CD, et al. 1987). The precise role and importance of these elements in the pathogenesis of osteoporosis are largely unknown.

Besides these nutritional factors, smoking results in a decreased amount of bone, as does alcohol abuse. Finally certain medications, particularly corticosteroids and Al-containing antacids, reduce bone mass or cause increased excretory loss of calcium.

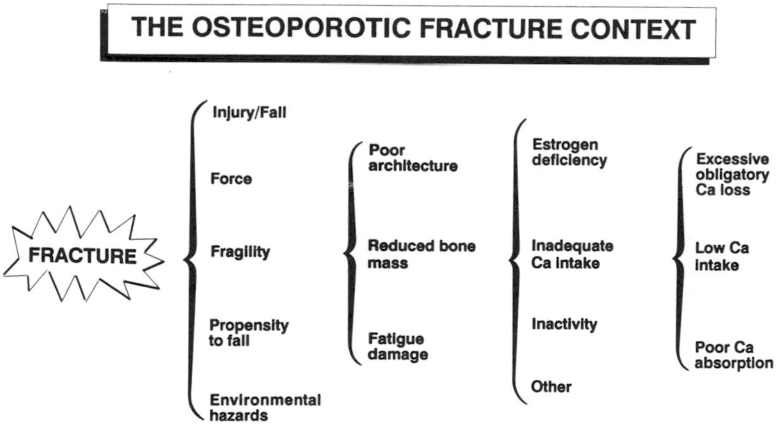

Fig. 2. The bone health and fragility context in which calcium nutrition is situated. Four major factors, arranged hierarchically, are involved: falls/injuries, fragility, mass, and nutrition. Each component listed has multiple contributing causes. For simplicity's sake, only the branch leading to calcium nutrition is developed. (Copyright, 1988, Robert P. Heaney. Used with permission.)

There is no easy way to be certain which of these factors is the cause in any given case of osteoporosis. Some women may be developing their osteoporosis primarily because of decreased physical activity, while others may be doing so because of decreased calcium intake, and yet others from silent alcohol abuse. Increasing calcium intake will not help the first very much, nor will increasing physical activity help the second. And nothing except temperance will help the third. It is because we cannot easily tell which is the main factor in any given case that it is important for all women to take such common sense measures as to assure good calcium intake throughout life, to maintain a vigorous program of physical activity, and to avoid excess use of alcohol and cigarettes.

Fig. 2 situates calcium nutrition in this larger context of bone health. Perhaps the best way to think about the issue is by way of analogy to anemia. Just as anemia is not a single disorder, with a single cause, neither is osteoporosis. Just as insufficient iron intake is but one of the causes of anemia, so insufficient calcium intake is but one of the causes of osteoporosis.

CALCIUM AND BONE HEALTH

Calcium is an essential nutrient for building and maintaining sound bones. This need has been recognized for many years and is shown clearly by the fact that low calcium diets regularly produce osteoporosis in experimental animals. But, as already noted, low calcium intake is not the only cause of osteoporosis.

While there is some controversy in regard to calcium intake and osteoporosis in humans, the disagreement concerns how little calcium is too little, not the basic relationship between calcium and bone health (Heaney RP 1988). The controversy has arisen because, even though most published studies have shown that increased calcium intake slows age-related bone loss, the effects have sometimes been undramatic, particularly when compared with the effects of ERT in early postmenopausal women. One reason is that women selected for studies of ERT are universally estrogen-deficient, whereas not all women given calcium in such studies have been calcium-deficient. (Such studies are like giving iron supplements to a group of unselected anemics. Some would respond, but of course others would not. The *average* change would thus usually be unimpressive.)

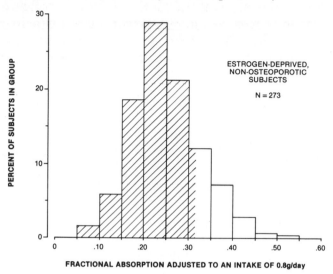

Fig. 3. Distribution of calcium absorption values in healthy early post-menopausal women, corrected to the current RDA (800 mg). The cross-hatched zone indicates absorption values below the minimum needed to offset minimum obligatory losses in typical U.S. women. As is evident, fully three-fourths are not absorbing enough to sustain calcium balance. (Copyright, 1988, Robert P. Heaney. Used with permission.)

Also, there is a wide variation among women in ability to adapt to a low calcium diet (Heaney RP and Recker RR 1986). By increasing absorption efficiency and reducing excretory losses, some women adapt perfectly well to low calcium diets. But others do not. Fig. 3 illustrates the range of absorptive performance in ostensibly healthy, early post-menopausal women, adjusted to a calcium intake of 800 mg/day. At this intake, absorption must be at least 32 percent to offset typical excretory losses. Less than one-fourth of these normal women were able to achieve that level of absorption efficiency.

Relatively high intakes of both protein and sodium may be a part of the explanation for poor adaptation, for both factors increase urinary loss of calcium. It seems likely that this is one of the reasons why First World women have higher calcium requirements than Third World women. Another reason is the increased prevalence of Vitamin D deficiency in middle-aged and elderly women. This is due in part to decreased solar exposure, partly to sluggish synthesis of calcitriol in the elderly, and partly to a blunted intestinal mucosal response to calcitriol in some osteoporotics. It is probably mainly for these reasons that utilization of dietary calcium is often inefficient in older women.

RECOMMENDED CALCIUM INTAKE

It is not easy to distinguish women who cannot adapt to low calcium intakes from others who can. In fact, there is no sure test for the recognition of calcium deficiency since, so long as parathyroid function is adequate, plasma calcium remains entirely normal, even on calcium-free intakes. Because some people clearly need more calcium than others, and because high calcium intakes are quite safe for the majority of people, it makes preeminently good sense to assure that every woman receive an adequate calcium intake.

This conclusion was reflected in the report of the 1984 NIH Consensus Conference on Osteoporosis, which recommended 1000 mg Ca/day for estrogen-replete perimenopausal women and 1500 mg Ca/day for estrogen-deprived postmenopausal women (Consensus Conference Statement on Osteoporosis 1984). These recommendations are entirely consistent with our own experience with perimenopausal women at Creighton University where, in over 500 studies, we have found significantly better calcium balance at higher intakes than at low (Heaney RP 1988). Our estimates of mean calcium requirement are precisely in the range of the NIH recommendations.

Although not all published studies have been able to show a significant relationship between calcium intake and bone mass, most have, and even a recent report from Denmark, widely interpreted in the public media as showing no effect of calcium, illustrates this point (Riis B, Thomsen K, et al. 1987). In brief, recently postmenopausal Danish women receiving a basal intake averaging nearly 1000 mg Ca/day, were nevertheless able to reduce bone loss when given additional calcium. This result showed that an average intake of 1000 mg/day was not enough to assure that calcium deficiency will not be contributing to age-related bone loss in some members of the population.

FOOD VS. PILLS

The preferable source of calcium is food, mainly naturally Ca-rich foods such as dairy products. There are many reasons for this preference. Most obvious is the fact that supplements can contain only the nutrients we know about. By contrast foods - being the healthy tissues of plants or animals - necessarily contain the nutrients required for their own health. For that reason they are more likely than are fabricated supplements to contain the nutrients necessary for our health as well. A recent example of that point is found in the still unconfirmed report, mentioned earlier, of the beneficial effect of boron on calcium metabolism and bone health (Nielsen FH, Hunt CD, et al. 1987). Up till the time of that report, it had not been known that boron had nutritional significance for humans. The point is, boron is relatively abundant in healthy fruit and vegetable foods, and so people eating those foods had been getting the mineral whether or not nutritionists knew they needed it.

Second, single nutrient supplements have a tendency to create imbalances of other nutrients, particularly some that may already be in marginal supply. Thus, large calcium supplements are known to interfere with iron absorption. This will not be a problem for everyone, but it illustrates the difficulty inherent in trying to manage nutrition with pills.

Third, though calcium is about as safe a supplement as one can find. Still, it is possible to take too many tablets, and for toddlers or children to overdose. That kind of toxicity is not possible with food sources.

Finally, osteoporosis is a complicated group of disorders, with many roots throughout a woman's lifestyle. Encouraging the idea that one can counteract a bad lifestyle with a pill is not good health policy.

FOOD FORTIFICATION

One of the problems an affluent society faces is a great reduction in personal energy expenditure. Correspondingly, we have had to cut back on calorie intake. This usually means a reduction in intake of many essential nutrients. To make matters worse, while total nutrient intake has been falling, our affluence has allowed us to increase our intake of empty calories (principally fat, sugar, and alcohol). The result is a further decline in several essential nutrients. One of these is calcium. Thus it seems important to increase the calcium nutrient density of various items in the food chain, just as, for many years, we have found it prudent to add iron and B vitamins to white bread.

Calcium-fortified foods can provide a valuable alternative calcium source for persons who will not get enough calcium from naturally high calcium foods (principally dairy products). However, some caution is in order in this regard, because simply adding calcium to a food does not guarantee its availability. Each additive needs to be tested in the food it is intended to fortify (Heaney RP 1986).

CALCIUM SUPPLEMENTS

Though food is better, still calcium supplements will be necessary for some women, such as those who are being treated for osteoporosis. High calcium intakes are a necessary component of all major osteoporosis treatment regimens. Because absorption efficiency tends to be even poorer in an osteoporotic woman than in a healthy woman her age, intakes in excess of 1500 mg/day are usually indicated. So a question frequently arises: which form of calcium is best, and when and how should it be taken?

The answers are not all known, but several principles seem applicable:

¤ Select a form that requires the least number of pills per day; compliance will be better that way.

¤ Select a form that is economical. Some of the very high cost supplements on the market have doubtful value in the first place (e.g., chelated calcium), and are certainly no more readily available than lower cost products.

¤ Choose a reliable manufacturer whose product has been tested and shown to be available. Many tablets are so poorly formulated that they do not break up in the stomach (Shangraw R 1988). They may be chemically identical to other products, but that is not the important factor. It is a matter of pharmaceutical formulation. Chewable tablets have a clear edge in that regard, since they necessarily break up before they are swallowed.

It is probably best to take calcium supplements with meals, both because absorption is slightly better that way (Heaney RP, Smith KT, et al. 1988), and because, when taken on an empty stomach, some women will malabsorb calcium carbonate and calcium phosphate (the two principal supplement forms on the market today). Many physicians recommend taking a calcium supplement at bedtime, with the theory being that doing so protects the bones during the night (when calcium is not being absorbed from food). That rationale makes preeminently good sense for most people. But it probably doesn't work for those few women who cannot absorb these products well on an empty stomach.

REFERENCES

Aaron JE, Makins NB, and Sagreiya K (1987). The microanatomy of trabecular bone loss in normal aging men and women. Clin Orthop Rel Res 215:260-271.

Carter DR, Caler WE, Spengler DM, and Frankel VH (1981). Fatigue bahavior of adult cortical bone: the influence of mean strain and strain range. Acta Orthop Scand 52:481-490.

Consensus Conference Statement on Osteoporosis (1984). JAMA 252:799-802.

Heaney RP (1986). Osteoporosis - the need and opportunity for calcium fortification. Cereal Foods World 31:349-353.

Heaney RP (1988). The calcium controversy: Finding a middle ground between the extremes. Public Health Reports (in press).

Heaney RP and Recker RR (1986). Distribution of calcium absorption in middle-aged women. Am J Clin Nutr 43:299-305.

Heaney RP, Smith KT, Recker RR, and Hinders SM (1988). Meal effects on calcium absorption. A J Clin Nutri (in press).

Kleerekoper M, Feldkamp LA, Goldstein SA, Flynn MJ, and Parfitt AM (1987). Cancellous bone architecture and bone strength. In Christiansen C, Johansen JS, et al. (eds): "Osteoporosis 1987," Viborg, Denmark: Norhaven A/S, pp 294-300.

Nielsen FH, Hunt CD, Mullen LM, and Hunt JR (1987). Effect of dietary boron on mineral, estrogen, and testosterone metabolism in postmenopausal women. Proc Soc Exp Biol Med 1:394-397.

Riis B, Thomsen K, and Christiansen C (1987). Does calcium treatment prevent postmenopausal bone loss? A double-blind controlled clinical study. N Engl J Med 316:173- 177.

Shangraw R (1988). Nutrition/Exercise. Public Health Reports (in press).

Mineral Homeostasis in the Elderly, pages 127–140
© *1989 Alan R. Liss, Inc.*

CHANGES IN INTESTINAL CALCIUM ABSORPTION AND VITAMIN D
METABOLISM WITH AGE

H. James Armbrecht

Geriatric Research, Education, and
Clinical Center, St. Louis Veterans
Administration Medical Center,
St. Louis, Missouri 63125 and
Departments of Medicine and
Biochemisty, St. Louis University
School of Medicine, St. Louis,
Missouri 63104

INTRODUCTION

Serum calcium (Ca) must be closely maintained
throughout the lifespan at about 10 mg/dl for the proper
function of nerve, muscle, and bone. Serum Ca is maintained primarily through the absorption of dietary Ca by
the intestine and the resorption of mineral Ca from bone.
The two major hormones involved in the regulation of Ca
metabolism are 1,25-dihydroxyvitamin D ($1,25(OH)_2D$), the
active metabolite of vitamin D, and parathyroid hormone
(PTH) (DeLuca, 1979; Henry, 1984). When serum Ca decreases
from its normal level, the parathyroid glands sense this
decrease and secrete PTH in proportion to the magnitude of
the fall. In younger animals, PTH acts on bone to increase
Ca resorption, and PTH also acts on the kidney to increase
the conversion of 25-hydroxyvitamin D to $1,25(OH)_2D$.
$1,25(OH)_2D$ increases the efficiency of Ca absorption by the
small intestine, and it also works in conjunction with PTH
to enhance bone resorption. These combined actions of
$1,25(OH)_2D$ and PTH on intestine and bone raise serum Ca
levels back to normal.

The mechanisms resposible for maintaining serum Ca
change with age in both rats and humans. In particular,
both species show a marked age-related decline in the
capacity of the small intestine to absorb dietary Ca. As a

result, the bone plays a greater role in the maintenance of serum Ca with advancing age. This increased role, along with age-related changes in bone and its hormonal regulators, may contribute to the decreased bone mass seen in the elderly.

Since the decrease in intestinal Ca absorption with age may alter Ca metabolism in the elderly, it is important to understand the mechanisms responsible for this decrease. We and others have used the rat as an animal model in which to study these mechanisms at the biochemical level. In addition, we have also studied age-related changes in vitamin D metabolism, since intestinal absorption is modulated by the vitamin D status of the animal.

This chapter is divided into three sections. In the first section, we will discuss the age-related changes in Ca absorption by the small intestine and their biochemical basis. In the second section, the evidence for a decline in serum $1,25(OH)_2D$ with age will be reviewed. In the last section, the role of the kidney in the decreased serum $1,25(OH)_2D$ levels will be addressed.

CHANGES IN INTESTINAL CA ABSORPTION WITH AGE

Ca Absorption in Humans

Several human studies have demonstrated that there is a decrease in the absorption of Ca with age (Alevizaki et al., 1973; Avioli et al., 1965; Bullamore, 1970). The precise relationship of the decrease to chronological age is uncertain due to the variability of clinical studies. One study reported that Ca absorption declined as a decaying exponential function of age (Alevizaki et al., 1973). Another study, using different experimental techniques, fit their data to a straight line (Avioli et al., 1965). However, this data could also have been fit to a decaying exponential. A third study, which examined an older population, reported a decrease in absorption after 60 years of age (Bullamore et al., 1970).

Ca Absorption in Rats

Ca absorption by rat small intestine, as measured by
everted intestinal segments, also declines with age. This
decline is most evident in the proximal duodenum. In
everted duodenal segments, active transport of Ca, as
measured by the S/M ratio, declines exponentially with age
(Figure 1) (Armbrecht et al., 1979; Armbrecht et al.,
1980c; Horst et al., 1978). The S/M ratio is the ratio of
Ca on the outside (serosa) of the sac to Ca on the inside
(mucosa) of the sac after a 1.5 hour incubation. The
incubation begins with equal amounts of Ca on both sides.
This technique measures primarily active, energy-dependent
Ca absorption.

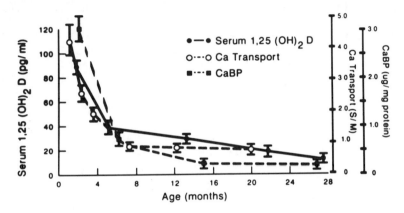

Figure 1. Changes in calcium and vitamin D metabolism with
age in F344 rats. Ca transport was measured using everted
duodenal sacs. Intestinal CaBP content was measured
immunologically. Serum 1,25-dihydroxyvitamin D was
measured by competitive binding assay. Data points are the
mean ± SEM of 4-8 rats.

Duodenal uptake of Ca also declines with age
(Armbrecht, 1986). To measure Ca uptake, everted
intestinal segments are incubated with Ca on the mucosal
side only for 15 minutes. Ca uptake into the mucosa is
quantitated and expressed per wet weight of tissue. Using
this technique, there is a 50% decrease in Ca uptake between 2-3 and 12 months of age with little further decrease
thereafter. This is similar to the decline in S/M ratio

with age (Figure 1). No age-related changes in Ca uptake were seen in the jejunum and ileum using this technique.

Mechanism of Intestinal Ca Absorption

A possible model for the active transport of Ca across the intestinal epithelial cell is shown in Figure 2 (Wasserman et al., 1984). Luminal Ca crosses the brush border membrane and enters the cell via a carrier-mediated process. This entry is probably passive, since the luminal Ca concentration is much higher than the intracellular concentration. Entry may be facilitated by a particulate Ca-binding complex (CaBC), which has been described (Kowarski and Schachter, 1980). Ca then moves across the absorptive cell to the basal lateral membrane. The cytosolic vitamin D-dependent Ca-binding protein (CaBP) may play a role in the translocation of Ca. This protein binds Ca with a high affinity, is markedly stimulated by $1,25(OH)_2D$, and correlates well with Ca absorption (Wasserman and Fullmer,

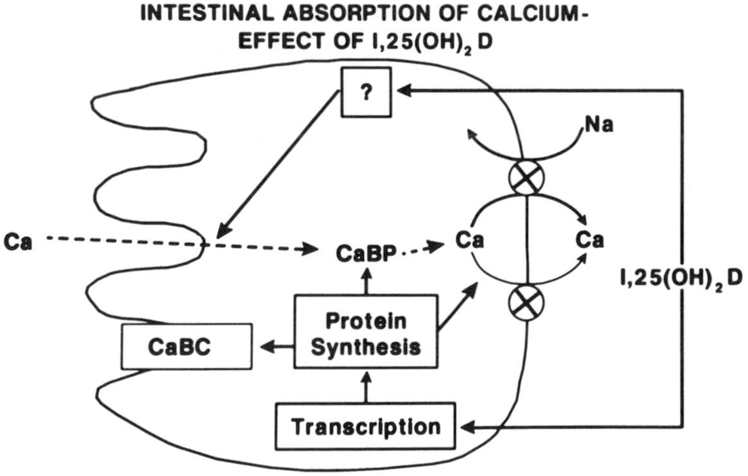

INTESTINAL ABSORPTION OF CALCIUM-
EFFECT OF $1,25(OH)_2D$

Figure 2. Effect of 1,25-dihydroxyvitamin D on intestinal absorption of calcium. CaBP and CaBC stand for intestinal calcium-binding protein and calcium-binding complex, respectively. See text for details.

1983). At the basal lateral membrane, Ca is actively pumped out of the cell. This is accomplished primarily by an ATP-dependent Ca pump (Ghijsen et al., 1982), with some contribution by a Na/Ca exchange mechanism.

1,25(OH)$_2$D acts at several sites to stimulate Ca absorption in young animals. 1,25(OH)$_2$D acts at the brush border membrane to enhance Ca entry into the cell. This action may involve alteration in the lipid composition of the membrane and increases in the CaBC (Kowarski and Schachter, 1980). In the cytoplasm, 1,25(OH)$_2$D increases the amount of CaBP, and increased CaBP may facilitate the movement of Ca across the cell (Wasserman and Fullmer, 1983). At the basal lateral membrane, 1,25(OH)$_2$D increases the capacity of the basal lateral membrane to actively pump Ca out of the cell (Ghijsen and Van Os, 1982). The long term effects of 1,25(OH)$_2$D are mediated by transcription and new protein synthesis.

Changes in Components of the Ca Transport System with Age

Using subcellular preparations, possible changes in components of the Ca transport system with age have been investigated. Ca movement across the brush border and basal lateral membranes were studied using isolated membrane vesicles, and CaBP concentrations was measured immunologically.

Using basal lateral membrane vesicles from the proximal duodenum, we found that there is a decrease in the capacity of vesicles to actively pump Ca with age. Vesicles isolated from 12 month old rats have a fivefold decrease in their capacity to actively pump Ca compared to 2 month old rats (Armbrecht and Doubek, 1987). There is no change in the passive (ATP-independent) component of Ca uptake with age. Kinetic studies show that the adult basal lateral membrane has a fivefold decrease in the number of Ca transporters (Vmax) but no change in transporter affinity (Km). The marked decrease in vesicle Ca uptake between 2 and 12 months correlates with the decrease in Ca active transport (Figure 1) and Ca uptake seen in the intact tissue.

The concentration of CaBP also declines markedly with age (Figure 1) (Armbrecht et al., 1979; Armbrecht et al.,

1980c). The concentration of this protein in the proximal duodenum was quantitated immunologically using antiserum provided by Dr. Elizabeth Bruns (University of Virginia, Charlottesville, VA). There is a large decrease in the concentration of CaBP between 2 and 6 months of age, followed by a slight decrease thereafter. These changes in CaBP closely parallel the age-related decrease in active transport seen in everted duodenal sacs (Figure 1).

In contrast to the basal lateral membrane, no age-related differences were seen in studies of Ca uptake by brush border membrane vesicles (Armbrecht, 1988). However, the Ca taken up by brush border membrane vesicles in these studies is not released by osmotic shock, as is Ca taken up by basal lateral membrane vesicles. This suggests that most of the Ca uptake by brush border membrane vesicles represents binding to the membrane itself rather than transport into the vesicular space. Such binding could mask age-related changes in Ca movement across the membrane. New experimental methods, which distinguish Ca binding from Ca movement across brush border vesicles, are needed to study this question.

CHANGES IN SERUM 1,25-DIHYDROXYVITAMIN D WITH AGE

One possible explanation for the decline in intestinal absorption of Ca is that there is a decrease in serum $1,25(OH)_2D$ with age. Another possibility is that there is a decrease in intestinal responsiveness to $1,25(OH)_2D$ with age.

Serum 1,25-Dihydroxyvitamin D Levels in Humans

A large number of studies have reported that serum $1,25(OH)_2D$ levels decrease with age (Lund et al., 1980; Gallagher et al., 1979; Fujisawa et al., 1984; Manolagas et al., 1983). Some studies have reported large decreases in serum $1,25(OH)_2D$ levels in the first two years of life (Lund et al., 1980). Other studies, which have focused on older adults, have reported a decrease in serum $1,25(OH)_2D$ later in life, between 50 and 65 years of age (Gallagher et al., 1979; Fujisawa et al., 1984). Another study found that there was a linear decline in serum $1,25(OH)_2D$ in adults aged 23-94 (Manolagas et al., 1983). The magnitude of the decline in serum $1,25(OH)_2D$ levels has been reported to be as large as 75% (Lund et al., 1980), although most studies report a decline of about 50% with age. It may be that in humans there is a decline in serum $1,25(OH)_2D$ during early childhood and also a decline later in life.

Serum 1,25-Dihydroxyvitamin D Levels in Rats

In rats, serum $1,25(OH)_2D$ levels decline exponentially with age (Armbrecht et al., 1988; Gray and Gambert, 1982). Serum $1,25(OH)_2D$ was measured by a competitive binding assay. The greatest decrease in serum $1,25(OH)_2D$ is between 2 and 5 months of age with a slight decline thereafter (Figure 1).

When serum $1,25(OH)_2D$ levels are plotted along with Ca absorption and CaBP (Figure 1), all the parameters show a similar decrease with age. There is a major decrease between 1-2 months and 5-7 months, followed by a lesser decline between 5-7 and 20-27 months. One explanation for the concurrent decline of these parameters is that the decrease in serum $1,25(OH)_2D$ results in a parallel decrease in the vitamin D-dependent CaBP. The decrease in CaBP then results in a decrease in the absorption of Ca, assuming that CaBP is rate-limiting for Ca transport.

Intestinal Responsiveness to 1,25-Dihydroxyvitamin D

There have been several animal studies of the effect of $1,25(OH)_2D$ on Ca transport as a function of age (Horst et al., 1978; Armbrecht, 1986; Armbrecht et al., 1980b). $1,25(OH)_2D$ significantly increases duodenal Ca transport as measured by the everted sac technique in 12 month old rats as well as in 2-3 month old rats (Horst et al., 1978; Armbrecht et al., 1980b). The time course of responsiveness is the same in both age groups, but the older rats are never stimulated to the same levels of transport as the young rats. Likewise, $1,25(OH)_2D$ increases Ca uptake by duodenal segments from both young and adult rats, but the uptake levels in the adult are never stimulated to the levels seen in the young (Armbrecht, 1986). In the ileum, $1,25(OH)_2D$ significantly stimulates Ca uptake in young animals but not in adult animals.

In terms of CaBP, $1,25(OH)_2D$ administration significantly increases duodenal CaBP content in both 2 and 12 month old animals (Armbrecht et al., 1980b). The time course of the response, as well as the peak levels attained, are very similar in each age group. However, in the same experiments, Ca transport in response to $1,25(OH)_2D$ is much less in adult compared to the young. Thus, the defect in adult responsiveness to $1,25(OH)_2D$ does not lie in the induction of CaBP. Further studies of the $1,25(OH)_2D$ responsiveness of other components, such as the brush border and basal lateral membranes, are needed. Also of interest is a recent report that the number and function of intestinal $1,25(OH)_2D$ receptors are altered with age (Takamoto et al., 1988).

CHANGES IN RENAL 1,25-DIHYDROXYVITAMIN D PRODUCTION WITH AGE

Since serum $1,25(OH)_2D$ levels decline with age, it is of interest whether this decline is due to decreased production of $1,25(OH)_2D$ or increased catabolism. In the rat, there is a marked decline in renal production of $1,25(OH)_2D$ with age. This decline is seen in vitro when $1,25(OH)_2D$ production is measured using either isolated renal slices (Armbrecht et al., 1980a) or renal mitochondria (Ishida et al., 1987). The greatest decrease in renal $1,25(OH)_2D$ production is between 2-3 and 12 months of age with little decrease thereafter. This decline in production correlates with the fall in serum $1,25(OH)_2D$ seen in this age range (Figure 1). Measurement of the catabolism of $1,25(OH)_2D$ in various age groups is needed to determine if catabolism plays a role in the decline in serum $1,25(OH)_2D$ with age.

Regulation of Renal 1,25-Dihydroxyvitamin D Production

In young animals, renal $1,25(OH)_2D$ production is regulated by many factors, including PTH and Ca (Henry and Norman, 1984). PTH stimulates $1,25(OH)_2D$ production and extracellular Ca inhibits it. The action of PTH is mediated by cAMP and the phosphorylation of specific proteins (Figure 3). PTH binds to its plasma membrane receptor, stimulates adenylate cyclase activity, and increases intracellular levels of cAMP (Armbrecht et al.,

1984). Increased levels of cAMP activate the
cAMP-dependent protein kinase found in the cytoplasm
(Armbrecht et al., 1984). This results in the
dephosphorylation of renal ferredoxin, an iron-sulfur
protein component of the 1-hydroxylase enzyme complex, and
in an increase in $1,25(OH)_2D$ production (Siegel et al.,
1986). This dephosphorylation may be mediated by a
phosphatase enzyme which is activated by a protein kinase
(Li et al., 1985).

Regulation of I,25(OH)$_2$D Production by PTH and Ca

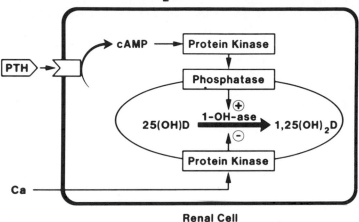

Renal Cell

Figure 3. Regulation of renal 1,25-dihydroxyvitamin D
production by PTH and calcium. See text for details.

Ca inhibits renal $1,25(OH)_2D$ production by a separate
pathway (Figure 3). The entry of Ca into the cell results
in the phosphorylation of renal ferredoxin and in an
inhibition of renal $1,25(OH)_2D$ production (Siegel et al.,
1986). This phosphorylation may be mediated by a
Ca-dependent protein kinase (protein kinase C) or other
components. The Ca and PTH pathways interact to regulate
$1,25(OH)_2D$ production. Extracellular Ca may moduluate the
stimulatory action of PTH (Fukase et al., 1984).

Effect of PTH on Renal 1,25-Dihydroxyvitamin D Production

There is evidence from both animal and human studies that PTH is less effective in stimulating $1,25(OH)_2D$ production in the old than in the young. In both rats and humans, serum PTH levels increase with age (Armbrecht et al, 1988; Gallagher et al., 1980) while serum $1,25(OH)_2D$ levels decrease. Administration of PTH to adult rats fails to stimulate $1,25(OH)_2D$ production, but PTH does stimulate $1,25(OH)_2D$ production in young rats (Armbrecht et al., 1982, Armbrecht et al., 1987). Interestingly, the refractoriness to PTH is specific, since administration of calcitonin to the adult animal significantly increases renal $1,25(OH)_2D$ production several fold (Armbrecht et al., 1987). In humans, renal responsiveness has been tested by infusing PTH into women of various ages (Tsai et al., 1984). The resulting increase in serum $1,25(OH)_2D$ in response to PTH declines with age. This suggests that the human kidney also becomes less responsive to PTH with age.

Recently, we have used isolated renal slices from rats of different ages to study this age-related response to PTH. Addition of PTH to renal slices from young rats stimulates $1,25(OH)_2D$ production in vitro (Armbrecht et al., 1982). However, PTH does not stimulate $1,25(OH)_2D$ production in renal slices from adult rats. Using renal slices, we have shown that the decreased responsiveness of the adult kidney is not due to decreased cAMP production or cAMP-dependent protein kinase activity (Armbrecht et al., 1986; Armbrecht and Scarpace, 1987). Rather, the decreased responsiveness may reflect altered phosphorylation of components of the renal 1-hydroxylase complex. We have recently shown that PTH does not alter the phosphorylation state of renal ferredoxin to the same extent in adult animals as in young animals (unpublished studies). The biochemical basis for this altered phosphorylation is currently under investigation.

SUMMARY

Intestinal absorption of Ca declines with age in both humans and rats. This decline in Ca absorption correlates with the age-related decline in serum $1,25(OH)_2D$ levels. At the cellular level, studies in rats suggest that the decline in serum $1,25(OH)_2D$ results in decreased levels of

CaBP and a decreased capacity of basal lateral membranes to actively pump Ca. Administration of $1,25(OH)_2D$ to older rats increases Ca absorption but not to the same levels seen in younger animals.

The age-related decrease in serum $1,25(OH)_2D$ levels may reflect decreased renal production of $1,25(OH)_2D$ with age. Decreased renal production, in turn, may reflect decreased renal responsiveness to PTH, since serum PTH levels rise with age in humans and rats. Studies in rats suggest that decreased renal responsiveness to PTH may be due to age-related changes in the phosphorylation of components of the 1-hydroxylase complex.

Hopefully, further studies will increase our knowledge of the mechanisms responsible for decreased Ca absorption by the intestine and decreased $1,25(OH)_2D$ production by the kidney with age. This knowledge may suggest new ways of enhancing Ca absorption, improving Ca balance, and decreasing bone loss in the elderly.

ACKNOWLEDGEMENTS

This research was supported by NIH grant AR32158 and by the Medical Research Service of the Veterans Administration. Appreciation goes to Cheryl Mason for preparation of this manuscript.

REFERENCES

Alevizaki CC, Ikkos DG, Singhelakis P (1973). Progressive decrease of true intestinal calcium absorption with age in normal man. J Nucl Med 14:760-762.
Armbrecht HJ (1986). Age-related changes in calcium and phosphorus uptake by rat small intestine. Biochim Biophys Acta 882:281-286.
Armbrecht HJ (1988). Changes in the components of the intestinal calcium transport system with age. In Bianchi L, Holt PR, James OFW, Butler RN (eds): "Aging in Liver and Gastrointestinal Tract," Lancaster, England: MTP Press, pp 131-139.
Armbrecht HJ, Boltz MA, Forte LR (1986). Effect of age on PTH and forskolin stimulated adenylate cyclase and protein kinase activity in the renal cortex. Exp

Gerontol 21:515–522.

Armbrecht HJ and Doubek WG (1987). Effect of age and lactose on calcium transport by intestinal basal-lateral membranes. Fed Proc 46:888.

Armbrecht HJ, Scarpace PJ (1987). Age-related changes in the adenylate cyclase system—Pharmacological and hormonal implications. In Wood WG, Strong R (eds): "Geriatric Clinical Pharmacology," New York: Raven Press, pp 179–188.

Armbrecht HJ, Strong R, Boltz M, Rocco D, Wood WG, Richardson A (1988). Modulation of age-related changes in serum 1,25-dihydroxyvitamin D and parathyroid hormone by dietary restriction. J Nutr, in press.

Armbrecht HJ, Wongsurawat N, Paschal R (1987). Effect of age on renal responsiveness to parathyroid hormone and calcitonin in rats. J Endocr 114:173–178.

Armbrecht HJ, Wongsurawat N, Zenser TV, Davis BB (1982). Differential effects of parathyroid hormone on the renal 1,25-dihydroxyvitamin D_3 and 24,25-dihydroxyvitamin D_3 production of young and adult rats. Endocrinology 111:1339–1344.

Armbrecht HJ, Wongsurawat N, Zenser TV, Davis BB (1984). Effect of PTH and 1,25(OH)D_3 on renal 25(OH)D_3 metabolism, adenylate cyclase, and protein kinase. Am J Physiol 246:E102–E107.

Armbrecht HJ, Zenser TV, Bruns MEH, Davis BB (1979). Effect of age on intestinal calcium absorption and adaptation to dietary calcium. Am J Physiol 236:E769–E774.

Armbrecht HJ, Zenser TV, Davis BB (1980a). Effect of age on the conversion of 25-hydroxyvitamin D_3 to 1,25-dihydroxyvitamin D_3 by the kidney of the rat. J Clin Invest 66:1118–1123.

Armbrecht HJ, Zenser TV, Davis BB (1980b). Effects of vitamin D metabolites on intestinal calcium absorption and calcium binding protein in young and adult rats. Endocrinology 106:469–475.

Armbrecht HJ, Zenser TV, Gross CJ, Davis BB (1980c). Adaptation to dietary calcium and phosphorus restriction changes with age. Am J Physiol 239:E322–E327.

Avioli LV, McDonald JE, Lee SW (1965). Influence of aging on the intestinal absorption of 47-Ca in women and its relation to 47-Ca absorption in postmenopausal osteoporosis. J Clin Invest 44:1960–1967.

Bullamore JR, Gallagher JC, Wilkinson R, Nordin BEC (1970). Effect of age on calcium absorption. Lancet ii:535–537.

DeLuca HF (1979). The vitamin D system in the regulation of calcium and phosphorus metabolism. Nutr Rev 37:161-193.

Fujisawa Y, Kida K, Matsuda H (1984). Role of change in vitamin D metabolism with age in calcium and phosphorus metabolism in normal human subjects. J Clin Endocrinol Metab 59:719-726.

Fukase M, Avioli LV, Birge SJ, Chase LR (1984). Abnormal regulation of 25-hydroxyvitamin D_3-1-alpha-hydroxylase activity by calcium and calcitonin in renal cortex from hypophosphatemic (Hyp) mice. Endocrinology 114:1203-1207.

Gallagher JC, Riggs BL, Eisman J, Hamstra A, Arnaud SB, DeLuca HF (1979). Intestinal calcium absorption and serum vitamin D metabolites in normal subjects and osteoporotic patients. J Clin Invest 64:729-736.

Gallagher JC, Riggs BL, Jerpbak CM, Arnaud CD (1980). The effect of age on serum immunoreactive parathyroid hormone in normal and osteoporotic women. J Lab Clin Med 95:373-385.

Ghijsen WEJM, De Jong MD, Van Os CH (1982). ATP-dependent calcium transport and its correlation with Ca-ATPase activity in basolateral plasma membranes of rat duodenum. Biochim Biophys Acta 689:327-336.

Ghijsen WEJM, Van Os CH (1982). 1,25-Dihydroxyvitamin D_3 regulates ATP-dependent calcium transport in basolateral plasma membranes of rat enterocytes. Biochim Biophys Acta 689:170-172.

Gray RW, Gambert SR (1982). Effect of age on plasma 1,25-$(OH)_2$ vitamin D in the rat. Age 5:54-56.

Henry HL, Norman AW (1984). Vitamin D: Metabolism and biological actions. Ann Rev Nutr 4:493-520.

Horst RL, DeLuca HF, Jorgenson NA (1978). The effect of age on calcium absorption and accumulation of 1,25-dihyroxyvitamin D in intestinal mucosa of rats. Metab Bone Dis Rel Res 1:29-33.

Ishida M, Bulos B, Takamoto S, Sacktor B (1987). Hydroxylation of 25-hydroxyvitamin D_3 by renal mitochondria from rats of different ages. Endocrinology 121:443-448.

Kowarski S, Schachter D (1980). Intestinal membrane calcium-binding protein. J Biol Chem 255:10834-10840.

Li H-C, Price DJ, Tabarini D (1985). On the mechanism of regulation of Type I phosphoprotein phosphatase from bovine heart. J Biol Chem 260:6416-6426.

Lund B, Clausen N, Lund B, Anderson E, Sorensen OH (1980).

Age-dependent variations in serum 1,25-dihydroxyvitamin D in childhood. Acta Endocrinol 94:426-429.

Manolagas SC, Culler FL, Howard JE, Brinkman AS, Deftos LJ (1983). The cytoreceptor assay for 1,25-dihydroxyvitamin D and its application to clinical studies. J Clin Endocrinol Metab 56:751-759.

Siegel NA, Wongsurawat N, Armbrecht HJ (1986). Parathyroid hormone stimulates dephosphorylation of the renoredoxin component of the 25-hydroxyvitamin D-1-alpha-hydroxylase from rat renal cortex. J Biol Chem 261:16998-17003.

Takamoto S, Liang T, Sacktor B (1988). Impaired DNA binding of intestinal 1,25(OH)$_2$D receptor in the aged rat. J Bone Mineral Res 3:S154.

Tsai KS, Heath H, Kumar R, Riggs BL (1984). Impaired vitamin D metabolism with aging in women. Possible role in pathogenesis of senile osteoporosis. J Clin Invest 73:1668-1674.

Wasserman RH, Armbrecht HJ, Shimura F, Meyer S, Chandler JS (1984). Vitamin D influences multiple phases of the intestinal calcium transport system. Prog Clin Biol Res 168:307-312.

Wasserman RH, Fullmer CS (1983). Calcium transport proteins, calcium absorption, and vitamin D. Ann Rev Physiol 45:375-390.

Mineral Homeostasis in the Elderly, pages 141–170
© *1989 Alan R. Liss, Inc.*

TRACE MINERAL REQUIREMENTS IN THE ELDERLY

Jeanne H. Freeland-Graves and Fares F. Behmardi

Graduate Nutrition Division, University of Texas at
Austin, Austin, Texas 78712

Specific nutrient requirements of essential trace elements for the elderly
have not been established. Currently, Recommended Dietary Allowances
(RDAs) have been set for zinc, iron, and iodine for adults, ages 23-50 and
51+ yrs (Food and Nutrition Board, 1980). For the next edition of the
RDAs, the adult categories for trace minerals have been proposed to be
divided as 25-50, 51-75, and 76+ yrs; however, these have not been
published to date. For other trace elements including copper, manganese,
fluoride, chromium, selenium, and molybdenum, Estimated Safe and
Adequate Daily Dietary Intakes (ESADDIs) have been formulated with
upper and lower suggested limits. These ranges are for all adults, with no
subcategories based on age.

This chapter will briefly review current knowledge regarding nutritional
status and requirements of the elderly for the following trace elements:
manganese, copper, zinc, iron, chromium, and molybdenum.

MANGANESE

Status

Only four studies have assessed manganese (Mn) status in the elderly.
In a 1983 Canadian study of post-menopausal women, Gibson et al.
compared 36 Seventh Day Adventist vegetarians (mean age = 69 yrs) to 30
nonvegetarians (mean age = 60.1 yrs) for manganese status as estimated
from levels in hair and 3-day diet records. Both hair (0.26 vs. 0.40 μg/g,
p< 0.003) and dietary intakes (2.6 vs. 4.4 mg/day, p< 0.005) were lower in
nonvegetarians than vegetarians, respectively. The higher intakes in
vegetarians were presumably due to the abundance of manganese in

legumes, nuts, and soy products. In the nonvegetarians, 43% had dietary levels less than the lower end of 2.5 - 5.0 mg/day range suggested by the Food and Nutrition Board (1980).

In a subsequent study of 90 free-living women (Gibson et al., 1985), aged 58-89 yrs (mean = 66.2 yrs), manganese levels in the diet averaged 3.8 mg/day and ranged from 1.6 to 11.2 mg. The large intakes in some subjects were related to a high consumption of tea, a beverage which is exceptionally rich in manganese. Low intakes (less than 2.5 mg) were found in 27% of the subjects.

A British study by Bunker et al. (1986) analyzed the manganese content of 35 different meals-on-wheels delivered to seven housebound elderly (mean age = 78.8 yrs). The meals contained an average of 10 µmol (0.5 mg) of manganese, which provided only 10% of the total amount, 81.9 µmol (4.5 mg), consumed for the day. The high level of the total intake was attributed to the large volumes of tea that were consumed.

Thus, tea appears to be a significant source of manganese in both Canadian and British diets. However, the bioavailability of the mineral in this beverage is subject to question. In a 1987 study, Kies et al. studied factors that affected manganese availability in ten human subjects. The addition of tea to the diet increased fecal excretion of manganese but did not improve its retention. The conclusion was that the polyphenols or other constituents in tea rendered the manganese unavailable for humans.

In the United States, an estimate of manganese in the diet was derived from analysis of 234 common foods (Pennington et al., 1986). Manganese levels in a typical diet were estimated as 2.12 mg/day for 60-65 yr women and 2.57 mg/day for 60-65 yr men.

Although postmenopausal women are not considered elderly, it is of interest to include the study by Hallfrisch et al. (1987) because of the limited data available on dietary manganese in older population groups in the United States. In this study, postmenopausal women, ages 49-65 yrs, donated duplicate samples of self-selected diets and all urinary and fecal excreta for 7 days. Analysis of the samples revealed that the women were consuming an average intake of 2.43 mg Mn/day, with a mean negative balance of -0.35 mg/day.

Masiak et al. (1981) measured manganese concentrations in the serum of 95 subjects, ages 20-93. Twenty-two percent of the samples were below the detectability of the method of analysis, i.e., neutron activation. No differences were seen for the different age groups, but males had significantly higher levels of serum manganese than did females. Ranges of serum manganese for 95% of the women were 0.01 to 0.70 µg/dl, and

0.01 to 0.73 µg/dl for the 95% of the men. It should be noted that serum manganese has been reported to be elevated in numerous disease states, including congestive heart failure, infection, and psychoses (Sullivan et al., 1979).

The only disease state in which serum manganese has been reported to be lowered is osteoporosis. The suggestion that manganese may be implicated in osteoporosis is derived from a 1986 study by Strause et al. Rats fed manganese-deficient diets for 12 months were reported to develop the same type of osteoporosis as that seen in a calcium deficiency. Manganese levels in serum and bone were depressed in conjunction with elevated serum calcium and phosphorus.

Elevations in serum calcium and phosphorus, as well as alkaline phosphatase activity, were also found in a human study by our laboratory (Friedman et al., 1987) in which seven males were fed a manganese-deficient diet (0.11 mg/day) for 39 days. The increases in these minerals in both humans and animals suggest that stores of manganese in bone were being mobilized as a consequence of a manganese depletion. Whether or not continued manganese depletion in humans would eventually lead to osteoporosis is an area which should be investigated more fully.

In 1987, a subsequent study by Strause and Saltman observed that serum levels of manganese in osteoporotic women were only 25% that of normal subjects. However, methods of analysis were not given and normal values of serum manganese presented in this paper are approximately forty times higher (0.04 mg/L or 40 µg/L) than that found in our laboratory (0.6 to 1.4 µg/L) (Freeland-Graves et al., 1988) when analyzed by graphite furnace atomic absorption spectrophotometry. This ambiguity makes it impossible to establish the relationship of manganese status to osteoporosis in humans. But in view of the high incidence of this disease in the elderly, future research in this area is imperative.

Requirements

The current estimated safe and adequate daily dietary for manganese is set at 2.5 - 5.0 mg/day (Food and Nutrition Board, 1980). This range was based on the study by McLeod and Robinson (1972) which found positive balances in four subjects consuming a diet that varied in manganese content from 2.48 to 3.15 mg/day. However, the diet consisted only of meat, ice cream, tea, coffee, and orange juice (in two subjects only).

A more recent study by the author calculated that the minimal requirement for manganese based on obligatory losses in young men consuming a semi-purified, Mn-deficient diet was 0.74 mg/day (Friedman et al., 1987). However, the contribution of unabsorbed manganese from the deficient diet could not be separated from endogenous losses even though the dietary intake was negligible (0.11 mg/day). In contrast, the requirement calculated may be artificially low since a deficiency state was induced. It is plausible that losses from bile and pancreatic secretions may decline during manganese depletion in an effort to maintain body stores. Thus, lower than normal values for endogenous losses may have occurred. This adaptation is a problem in all balance studies that use a deficiency diet to determine minimal nutrient requirements.

A subsequent study in our laboratory (Freeland-Graves et al., 1988) fed five males varying levels of manganese in a diet of conventional foods for 105 days. Negative retention was observed on the first three dietary levels fed (2.89, 2.06 and 1.21 mg Mn/day), but became positive when manganese was added back to the diet. The recommended intake of manganese as determined by regression analysis of intake versus metabolic balance when intake would theoretically be zero, combined with an average retention of 11%, suggested a level of 3.5 mg/day. This level exceeds the current lower level of the ESADDI of 2.5 mg.

Evidence that the 3.5 mg minimal level may be more appropriate than the current 2.5 mg value is given in a recent review by the authors (Freeland-Graves et al., 1987). In this paper, a recalculation of data derived from numerous manganese balance studies in the literature suggested a recommended range of 3.5 to 7 mg Mn /day for adult males. This level was based on regression analysis of manganese balance versus dietary intakes from 11 different studies that fed diets of conventional foods that did not exceed 11 mg Mn/day.

Although this recommendation is higher than that suggested by the Food and Nutrition Board (1980), numerous studies (Freeland-Graves et al., 1987) have reported that it is difficult to achieve positive balance on dietary intakes of less than 3.5 mg. For example, negative balance of manganese occurred when bran muffins were added to the diet despite a dietary level of 13.9 mg Mn/day (Schwartz et al., 1986). The detrimental influence of bran is related to its high concentration of both fiber and phytates, compounds which have been reported to interfere with plasma uptake of the mineral (Bales et al., 1987).

Another example is the study of postmenopausal women by Hallfrisch et al. (1987) in which subjects were fed a diet based on complex carbohydrates for 3 months. Negative balances were found when the manganese level was 4.35 mg/day and positive balances occurred at intakes of 6.18 mg.

One possible reason for the great number of negative balances on what have been assumed to be adequate dietary intake levels of manganese (Freeland-Graves et al., 1987) is the influence that dietary factors have on manganese. Both animal and human studies have reported that calcium (Lin and Freeland-Graves, this volume; McDermott and Kies, 1987), iron (Dougherty et al., 1987; Gruden 1977), fiber, phytates (Bales et al., 1987), and sugar (Hallfrisch et al., 1987) have a detrimental effect on either the absorption or retention of the mineral. Thus, the current lower level of 2.5 mg/day for the ESADDI may be too low to maintain positive balance because of interacting effects of other dietary components.

The only other country that has also established a recommended intake for manganese is the U.S.S.R. Since their recommended range is 5 - 10 mg/day (Truswell, 1983), our suggestion of a range of 3.5 - 7 mg/day does not seem so unreasonable.

However, specific recommendations for advanced age cannot be made since there are no studies of manganese balance in the elderly. This gap in manganese requirements of the elderly suggests an urgent need for future research in this area.

COPPER

Status

Dietary intakes of copper (Cu) in the elderly have been found in several studies to be well below levels recommended for optimal health. Daily copper intakes of populations older than age 60 have averaged 0.69 mg (Bunker et al., 1986), 0.85 mg (Bunker et al., 1987) and 1.28 mg (Bunker et al., 1984) in the United Kingdom; 0.86 and 1.17 mg for males and females, respectively, in the United States (Pennington et al., 1986); 1.15 mg in Sweden (Abdulla, 1986); 1.2 mg (Gibson et al., 1985) and 1.6 mg (Gibson et al., 1983) in Canada; and 2.1 mg in Australia (Baghurst and Record, 1987). The lowest dietary intakes are associated with high levels of copper in plasma and whole blood and lower levels in leukocytes (Bunker et al., 1987).

Serum levels of copper have been found to increase with advancing age (Masiak et al., 1981; Harman et al., 1965; Bunker et al., 1984a), but this has been disputed (Vir et al., 1979). Yunice et al. (1974) observed that only males exhibited this increase, which was small. The relationship of endogenous and exogenous (i.e., oral contraceptives) hormones to this lack of change in females is unclear.

Harman et al. (1965) suggested that the high copper levels may be related to the free radical theory of aging. It was postulated that the mineral may act as an oxidation catalyst in the reduction of molecular oxygen. Increased concentration of ionized copper could increase peroxidation which eventually could lead to biochemical alterations that are associated with aging. In healthy elderly, the reported increase in serum copper has not been associated with other parameters of copper status such as ceruloplasmin (Yunice et al., 1974) or leukocyte copper (Bunker et al., 1984a). The failure of an increase in ceruloplasmin when serum copper increases suggests an elevation in either the ionized form or that bound to amino acids. Further study is needed to clarify the form of increased copper. Serum copper levels have also been shown to be elevated in congestive heart failure, infection, psychoses (Sullivan et al., 1979), malignancies (Lindeman, 1986), and periodontal disease (Freeland and Cousins, 1976).

Two studies have investigated tissue concentrations of copper in aging. Shroeder et al. (1966) found that copper concentrations in the aorta and liver decline after age 60; whereas, levels in heart, kidney, spleen and brain are the same. Taylor et al. (1974) also found that copper concentrations in coronary arteries decline with age as the lipid fraction increases. This reported decline of copper content in the aorta is undesirable since studies (O'Dell et al., 1961; Shields et al., 1962) have reported that copper deficiency leads to aneurysms and other cardiovascular lesions.

A concern regarding copper status in the elderly may be the widespread use of high-dose nutritional supplements. A survey of 270 free-living elderly (>60 yr) found that approximately 60% used nutritional supplements. Ascorbic acid was the most popular type. Mean supplemental intake of ascorbic acid was 570% of the Recommended Dietary Allowance for women and 830% for men (Garry et al., 1982). Another study in a retirement community (Gray et al., 1983) reported that 67% of a population of 51 subjects were taking ascorbic acid supplements. The median intake was 505 mg ascorbic acid/day, ranging from 30 to 5,200 mg. These high doses may have an adverse effect on copper status according to a study by Finley et al. (1983). In 13 young men, consumption of 1,500 mg ascorbic acid supplements for 2 months increased serum copper levels and reduced ceruloplasmin activity. Whether this antagonistic effect of ascorbic acid on copper status is also true in the elderly deserves to be explored.

High dose supplements of zinc may also affect copper status. In the survey of elderly by Garry et al. (1982), 31% of the males and 24% of the females used zinc supplements. Festa et al. (1985) found that dietary intakes of 18.5 mg/day reduced copper retention after one week, even with a dietary copper intake of 2.6 mg/day, In contrast, Taper et al. (1980) reported that varying the zinc levels of the diet as 8, 16 and 24 mg/day had no influence on copper retention in adult females. However, negative copper balance occurred on all three zinc levels despite a copper intake of 2 mg/day. It is possible that this failure of zinc to influence copper retention may be related to poor absorbability of the inorganic salt rather than total dietary levels.

The level of protein is another factor that may alter copper status. In balance studies lasting for periods of 2 to 24 months, Sandstead (1982a) reported that the copper requirement was highest when the level of dietary zinc is high and the protein is low. Thus, individuals habitually consuming such diets have an increased risk of copper deficiency. Increasing the level of protein at the same dietary zinc level decreases the requirement.

Finally, the source of dietary carbohydrate may also affect copper status. In 1987, Hallfrisch et al. found that switching the complex carbohydrates in a diet to create one high in simple sugars produced negative balances of the mineral due to increased fecal excretion. A detrimental effect of simple sugars on copper status has previously been found in rats (Reiser et al., 1983). Since the elderly have been reported to choose foods that are high in refined carbohydrates (Albanese et al., 1976), i.e., sucrose and dextrose, copper requirements could be elevated by such a diet. Other factors that may increase the copper requirement are the presence of cadmium and dietary fiber and phytate.

Requirements

The current safe and adequate range of copper of 2-3 mg/day (Food and Nutrition Board, 1980) is based on a limited number of studies conducted in the 1970's. Equilibrium or slightly positive balances were found when New Zealand women (Robinson et al., 1973) and preadolescent girls (Price et al., 1970) were fed diets containing copper levels ranging from 1.55 to 2.09 mg/day. In 1974, a minimal requirement of 1.65 mg/day for adults was determined by Hartley et al. Thus, the range of 2-3 mg of Cu/day was established to provide a margin of safety.

Since that time, a number of other studies have appeared. An exhaustive review of the literature by Mason (1979) concluded that levels of 1-2 mg Cu/day were sufficient to maintain positive balance in adults. In 1980, a metabolic ward study by Klevay et al. estimated a copper requirement of 1.55 mg/day based on typical diets consumed in the United States. The 1.55 mg was derived from the results of a linear regression equation of fecal and urinary losses of 1.30 mg/day, combined with an estimate of surface losses of 0.25 mg/day. A more recent review by Sandstead (1982a) suggested a slightly higher range, from 1.5 to 2 mg Cu/day.

A study by Shike et al. (1981) measured copper balance in 28 patients, ages 15-73 yrs, who were receiving total parenteral nutrition. A requirement of 0.3 mg/day was determined for patients with normal gastrointestinal excretion. The requirement increased to 0.4 to 0.5 mg/day in patients with increased fluid loss through diarrhea, gastrointestinal stomas or fistulas. These values, however, reflect endogenous losses only, and do not take into account possible inhibitory factors in a diet of conventional foods.

A number of metabolic balance studies of copper have been conducted in the elderly. The first one was by Wester (1971) who measured balance in two older men who were hospitalized for pancreatic insufficiency. One patient consuming 1.6 mg Cu/day was in positive balance, while a second patient receiving 0.98 mg Cu/day was in negative balance. If the three elderly patients (>60 yr) consuming a constant diet in the study by Hartley et al. (1974) are examined separately, a mean intake of 1.83 mg/day produced a positive balance of 0.41 mg.

Burke et al. (1981) conducted copper balance studies in elderly subjects, ages 56-83 yrs, who were fed a diet of conventional foods. The diet containing 1.05 mg Cu/day was supplemented with copper sulfate to achieve a total intake of 2.33 mg/day. But only fecal losses were used to calculate retention. When dietary zinc intakes were low (7.8 mg/day), mean copper retention was three times (0.94 vs. 0.30 mg) the level compared to when dietary zinc intakes were high (23.3 mg/day). Thus, excess zinc can adversely affect copper balance, as has been shown in younger subjects (Greger et al., 1978). However, a copper intake of 2.33 mg/day was sufficient for positive balance except in two individuals on the high zinc regimen.

In a study by Turnlund et al. (1981), copper balances were measured in 10 males between the ages of 65 and 75 yrs. A semi-purified formula diet was fed that varied in nitrogen (N) as either 9 to 19 mg/day or 70 mg N/kg body weight. The copper intakes of 3.24 and 3.28 mg/day for two separate 6-week periods produced positive balances of 0.01 and 0.06 mg/day, respectively. But no estimate was made for surface losses which could markedly affect balance. One subject in the first study and three subjects in the second study were in negative balance. The subject who was in negative balance both times had increased serum copper at the end of the study, suggesting that his status was less than optimal at the beginning. The mean [65]Cu absorption in seven of the subjects (Turnlund et al., 1982b) was 25.8% and an average of 0.85 mg Cu was absorbed from the 3.3 mg daily intake. The conclusions were that the levels of copper fed were sufficient to maintain balance in elderly men. However, the requirement for copper seemed to be more near the upper end of the ESADDI.

Two studies by Bunker et al. measured copper balances in the elderly consuming their self-selected diets for 5 days. In the first study (1984) of 24 healthy elderly (69-85 yrs), the mean dietary intake of copper was 1.28 mg/day, ranging from 0.65 to 3.04 mg in women and 0.84 to 2.3 mg in men. The mean copper retention was based on urinary and fecal losses and averaged -0.05 mg/day, ranging from -0.56 to 0.40 mg/day. Compared to an earlier study in the same laboratory (Aggett et al., 1983), both intakes and retention of copper was lower in the elderly compared to children. However, the elderly showed no signs of copper deficiency.

In the second study by Bunker et al. (1987), 20 housebound elderly (70-85 yr) with stable chronic diseases were compared to the healthy elderly above (Bunker et al., 1984). Dietary intakes of copper were low in the housebound elderly, averaging 0.85 mg/day, and ranged from 0.44 to 2.84 mg in the women and from 0.54 to 1.84 mg in the men. Reasons for the low intakes were related to reduced energy requirements due to decreased physical activity and ill health rather than poor nutrient density. The subjects had an average negative retention of 0.11 mg/day as measured from fecal and urinary losses. The addition of surface losses would make this figure even more negative. Parameters of copper status were also low.

The copper content of self-selected diets of 12 post-menopausal women (49-65 yrs) were also low in the study by Hallfrisch et al. (1987). A self-selected dietary level of 1.05 mg/day produced a mean negative balance of 130 µg/day. When subjects began consuming a prepared diet high in complex carbohydrates for 12 weeks, the intakes rose to 1.54 mg Cu/day and the balance became positive (60 µg).

The above studies suggest that the recommended intake of 2-3 mg seems to be adequate for most healthy elderly and that the actual level needed might be near the upper range. However, a number of elderly are consuming diets that fall far below this level. Consumption of these low levels, coupled with a high sugar intake and use of ascorbic acid and zinc supplements, may lead to significant problems in maintaining optimal copper nutriture.

ZINC

Status

Daily mean dietary intakes of zinc (Zn) have been reported to average 5.85 mg in British housebound elderly (Bunker et al., 1987); 7.5 mg in American postmenopausal women (Hallfrisch et al., 1987); 12.64 and 8.51 mg in elderly American men and women, respectively (Pennington et al., 1986); 8.96 mg in British healthy elderly (Bunker et al., 1984a); 11.2 and 12.4 mg in the Health and Nutrition Examination I (HANES I) (DHEW, 1979) and NHANES II (DHEW, 1981) surveys, respectively, and 12.6 mg/day in free-living elderly Australians (Baghurst and Record, 1987).

None of these studies show that the average elderly individual is meeting the RDA for zinc. Since rampant zinc deficiencies are not apparent and most of the elderly in these studies were reported as healthy, it seems probable that the RDA for zinc may be higher than necessary. In fact, a comparison of the United States RDA for zinc with recommended levels from other countries shows that others have set levels that are more easily provided by typical diets (Truswell, 1983).

Using data from the 1977-1978 Nationwide Food Consumption Survey, the 1968-1970 Ten-State Nutrition Survey, and NHANES II, Sandstead et al. (1982b) concluded that zinc intakes were dependent on energy intakes. Therefore, other than income, a primary reason that zinc intakes may be low in the elderly is the decrease in energy requirements and hence, caloric intakes.

Zinc levels in plasma and serum have been reported to decline with advanced age. In a study of 1,416 subjects (ages 15 to 70+) in Finland, serum zinc declined with age (Bjorksten et al., 1978). The decline was more evident in males than females. In NHANES II, serum zinc was measured in 14,770 persons, ages 3 to 74 yrs (Pilch and Senti, 1984). A decline in serum zinc with age was found in males but not in females. In a study of 258 subjects between 20 to 84 yrs old (Lindemen et al. 1971), plasma zinc was found to be inversely related to age in both males and females. In contrast, others have found no such association (Flint et al., 1981; Vir et al., 1979; Wagner et al., 1980).

Other measurements of zinc in human tissues such as hair (Petering et al., 1971), bone (Alhava et al., 1977) and kidney (Schroeder et al., 1967) have also been reported to decline with advanced age. Wagner et al. (1981) found that hair zinc levels were lower in elderly women of lower socioeconomic status. In contrast, Schor et al. (1984) found no decline in bone zinc in an autopsy study of subjects aged 0.5 to 91 yrs. Also, no relationship of age to hair zinc was found by Greger and Sciscoe (1977).

It is unclear whether the reported decline in serum, plasma, or tissue zinc is a physiological consequence of aging or the result of a long-standing sub-optimal dietary intake. It should be mentioned that the parameters which have been measured, such as blood and hair, are not always reliable parameters of zinc status (Solomons et al., 1986). One parameter of zinc status, the plasma zinc uptake test, was found to be significantly lower in healthy elderly compared to young controls (Bales et al., 1986). The reader is referred to other chapters in this book (Solomons; Prasad; Greger) which more adequately discuss this area.

Although dietary intakes do fall far below the RDAs, most elderly appear to be in adequate zinc status. But since there are reports of very low dietary intakes and low zinc nutriture in some cases (Paterson et al., 1985; Bales et al., 1986), it is plausible that some elderly have potential problems in zinc nutrition.

Requirements

The current RDA of 15 mg is based on the study by Spencer et al. (1976) that found equilibrium or positive balance on a zinc intake of 12.5 mg/day. Since the daily turnover of radioisotopic zinc has been calculated to be 6 mg (Engel et al., 1966), an absorption of 40% was used to produce the 15 mg value. However, the figure of 40% has recently been questioned by the Food and Nutrition Board (1986).

Further evidence that the endogenous losses of zinc may be approximately 6 mg/day is presented in a study of patients receiving total parenteral nutrition (Wolman et al., 1979). This method may be used to estimate requirements since it has been reported that any excess zinc that is administered is retained and not excreted (Jeejeebhoy et al., 1986). Thus, the amount excreted as endogenous losses is assumed to be the absolute requirement.

The authors found only four groups of researchers who have conducted metabolic balance studies of zinc in older individuals. The first by Wester (1971) involved two men, 52 and 62 years old, who were hospitalized for pancreatic insufficiency. Dietary intakes that averaged either 9.7 or 16 mg Zn/day produced positive balances of 4.79 and 8.08 mg/day, respectively. In 1974, Hartley et al. conducted metabolic studies in patients hospitalized for a variety of bone and gastrointestinal disorders. In the patients who were >60 yrs and consuming a normal diet, one patient was in negative balance (-0.13 mg) on a daily zinc intake of 9.48 mg/day and two of the patients were in positive balance at intakes that were 15.04 to 16.42 mg/day.

In Great Britain, Bunker et al. compared dietary intakes and metabolic balances in 24 healthy (1984a) and 20 housebound (1987) elderly in Great Britain. Duplicate samples of diet and all excreta (feces and urine) were collected for 5 days and analyzed for zinc concentrations. In the report of 24 healthy elderly, zinc concentrations in the diets averaged 8.96 mg/day. Net retention was positive at 0.07 mg/day, but ranged from -3.08 to 2.03 mg/day. Body surface losses were not measured, but the addition of these would presumably make the retention less positive. Since these subjects showed no signs of a zinc deficiency despite dietary intakes that are 59% of the RDA, the authors concluded that good health can be maintained on this dietary level.

In the housebound elderly (Bunker et al., 1987), zinc intakes were much lower, averaging 5.85 mg/day. This low level of intake produced a mean negative balance of -1 mg/day. However, overt signs of zinc deficiency were not obvious in these subjects.

In the United States, Burke et al. (1981) measured the metabolic balance of zinc in 10 healthy elderly (56-83 yr) throughout a 30-day feeding study. The baseline diet of conventional foods contained an average of 6.03 mg zinc, which was supplemented with zinc sulfate to create two dietary zinc levels of either 7.80 or 23.3 mg/day. Half of the subjects on each dietary level were in negative balance. Integumental losses of zinc were not measured and the authors suggested that their inclusion would result in most of the subjects being in negative balance. The failure of 23.3 mg zinc intake to produce positive balance is surprising but was attributed to the possible poor absorption of a zinc supplement when given with foods.

Turnlund et al. (1981) measured zinc balances in six elderly males consuming varying levels of protein in the diet. On a zinc intake of 15.4 to 15.5 mg/day, a mean positive balance of 0.1 mg/day was reported. However, half of the subjects had mean negative balances and integumental and sweat losses were not included. Although body surface losses were measured, the contamination in blanks was too great for the data to be reliable. However, an estimate of a maximal surface loss of less than 0.5 mg for zinc was suggested. The addition of this 0.5 mg for surface losses would have made the balances negative. The authors concluded that balance studies are not sensitive enough to determine the impact of small deficiencies or increases over a long period of time.

In a subsequent paper, the absorption of radioactive zinc was compared in six elderly males to six young males (Turnlund et al., 1986). Although zinc balance did not vary between the groups, the old absorbed significantly less zinc from their diet, 17%, compared to the young, 31%. The lower absorption rates may suggest that elderly have lower zinc requirements for absorbed zinc than the young. One factor that might contribute to lower zinc requirements would be a decrease in sexual activity due to dysfunction since seminal losses of Zn can be as much as 0.5 mg per ejaculate (Truswell et al., 1986). Thus, a reduction in sexual activity could significantly lower the need for this mineral in males.

Another explanation could be that the decline in lean body mass that occurs with aging could lead to diminished endogenous losses. Hence, there would be less need to replace losses. Also, a decline in physical activity in the elderly would reduce endogenous losses through sweat. However, decreased physical activity is not necessarily associated with aging.

Whereas, Turnlund et al. reported zinc absorption in subjects eating semipurified diets, Aamodt (1983) used only fasting subjects. When zinc absorption was measured in 75 fasting subjects (ages 18 - 84 yrs), absorption averaged 65% and ranged from 40 to 86%. A significant correlation (r = - 0.93, p < 0.0001) was found between age and zinc absorption. The decline was estimated at approximately a tenth of a percent per year within the age range studied. Thus, both of the above studies have found decreased zinc absorption with advanced age.

In estimating requirements for dietary zinc, it is important to remember that the requirement will vary according to the bioavailability of the mineral. The World Health Organization (WHO, 1973) has formulated a provisional requirement of 22 mg/day when zinc is 10% available; this requirement declines to 11 mg/day when zinc is 20% available. An excellent review of how food factors, such as phytate, fiber, type of fat, nitrogen, tin and phosphate, influence the bioavailability of dietary zinc is recommended (Sandstead et al., 1982b). Although fiber has been reported to influence zinc balance (Smith et al., 1983), studies in pre- and postmenopausal women (Hallfrisch et al., 1987) and men aged 34 to 58 yr (Kelsay et al., 1983) did not find such an effect.

In summary, it is unclear whether or not the elderly have zinc requirements that differ from young adults. Some data suggest that the need for zinc may actually be lower for males if sexual activity declines. Confusion still exists as to whether the current 15 mg RDA for zinc for adults is set too high (Food and Nutrition Board, 1980) since few people consume this amount in their diets and evident zinc deficiency is not apparent in developed countries. But the fact that the absorption of zinc has been reported to decline with age suggest that the elderly may not be as adaptable as the young in maintaining adequate status on low intakes.

IRON

Status

The iron (Fe) status of the elderly in the United States has been the subject of several excellent reviews (Lynch et al., 1982; Nordstrom, 1982; Pilch and Senti, 1984). Lynch et al. reported that there were only a limited number of studies on iron status in the elderly, particularly for those over age 75. Up to this age, nutrition surveys have found that most Americans meet the dietary iron level of 10 mg set by the Food and Nutrition Board (1980). However, the possibility of altered bioavailability of iron from a reduced meat intake and an increase in the proportion supplied by breakfast cereals has not been studied. Although physiological indicators do not indicate any significant iron deficiency in most elderly, the incidence in disadvantaged population groups is not well known.

Nordstrom (1982) reviewed data from the Ten-State Nutrition Survey (CDC, 1972), the Missouri Nutrition Survey (Kohrs et al., 1978), the Nutrition program participants in Missouri (Kohrs et al., 1980), the HANES survey (DHEW 1979 and 1981) and a study of elderly in Boston (Gershoff et al., 1977). Anemia was prevalent more frequently in Blacks, and in individuals with lower incomes and advanced age, particularly for males. Lower mean hemoglobin levels found in Blacks were attributed, in part, to low dietary intakes of iron.

Although some of the above studies indicated a high incidence of anemia in the elderly, the type of anemia was not clarified. In 1984, Dallman et al. measured the prevalence and causes of anemia in the United States in 11,547 subjects who participated in the NHANES II survey. Anemia was present in 4.4% of elderly men, but the causes were believed to be related to inflammatory diseases rather than iron deficiency. It was suggested that age-specific reference standards be set for elderly men; whereas, the same set of standards can be used for anemia in women of all ages. Thus, most anemia in the elderly does not appear to be related to iron deficiency. The exception are some subgroups of the population such as elderly Blacks, particularly males, in which the prevalence of iron deficiency has been reported to be as high as 23% (Macarthy et al., 1987) and 50.3% (CDC, 1972). In addition to health and race, other factors that may be responsible for the high prevalence of anemia in past studies are socioeconomic status and region (Garry et al., 1983).

Others have found no evidence of impaired iron status in the elderly (Freedman and Ahronheim, 1985; Gershoff et al., 1977; Marx et al., 1979; Bailey et al., 1979). In fact, advanced age has been associated with increased iron stores, as indicated by serum ferritin (Casale et al., 1981; Cook et al., 1976; Loria et al., 1979; MacPhail et al., 1981) and liver iron (Loh and Chang, 1980). At all ages, males had higher stores than females. Whether or not increasing the iron stores of women would offer a greater protection against iron-deficiency anemia is unclear (Food and Nutrition Board, 1986). In contrast, Valberg et al. (1976) found no increase in iron stores after the age of 20.

Requirements

The current RDA for iron for males and females, age 51+, is 10 mg. In the next edition of the RDAs, the proposed values for adults age 51-75 and 76+ will remain at 10 mg. This figure is derived from studies that measured turnover of body iron. In 1959, Finch et al. conducted radioisotopic studies in which intravenously- administered ^{55}Fe was allowed to equilibrate for up to 54 months. The iron turnover of total misicible body iron estimated by this method averaged 0.61, 0.64, and 1.22 mg/day in men (57-84 yrs), nonmenstruating women (49-77 yrs) and menstruating women (32-44 yrs), respectively. This technique was also used by Green et al. (1968) who found slightly higher values of 0.90, 0.95, and 1.02 mg/day in Venezuelan Mestizo, Seattle Caucasian, and Durban Indian males, respectively. Thus, the average iron loss of adult males is approximately 1 mg/day.

The Food and Nutrition Board (1980) combined this average loss of 1 mg/day with an average absorption of 10% to produce the RDA for iron of 10 mg/day for adult males. The RDA for premenopausal adult females (age 23-50 yrs) is set higher, at 18 mg, to allow for menstrual losses. In the new RDAs, it is proposed that the level be set slightly lower, 15 mg. After menopause, the requirements for females would be similar to that of males since monthly blood losses terminate.

The average absorption of 10%, however, is subject to criticism since it will vary greatly according to the proportion of heme vs. nonheme iron, iron status of the individual and the presence of dietary ascorbic acid, meat, poultry, fish, tannic acid, phosvitin, phytates, calcium and phosphate salts, EDTA, and antacids (Monsen et al., 1976). It is now recommended that the quantity of absorbable iron be calculated when evaluating iron intake. Thus, 1.0 mg of *absorbable* iron is the recommended intake, but the dietary level needed to achieve this amount will vary.

Older studies reported that iron absorption decreased with age (Bonnet et al., 1960). However, these data are now considered questionable since the studies were not well controlled for iron status and the absence of a disease state (Lynch et al., 1982). For example, in a study by Jacob and Owens (1969), absorption of ^{59}Fe was less in older subjects (>50 yrs.) compared to younger subjects (<30 yrs.), 13.1 vs. 26%. No differences were seen in absorption of heme iron. The iron status of the subjects was assumed to be adequate as determined by serum iron and transferrin saturation. Yet these parameters are no longer considered definitive indices of iron status. Lower absorption rates in the older studies were suggested to be due to decreased gastric secretion (hydrochloric acid). But Lynch et al. (1982) has suggested that the lower rates could also be an inverse function of higher body stores.

Using dual isotopes, Marx et al. (1979) found that iron mucosal uptake (37.6 vs. 41.0%) and retention (20.0 vs. 25.3%) did not differ significantly between young (22-48 yr) and old (65-83 yr) males, respectively. However, an increase in ineffective erythropoiesis was suggested since the young utilized more iron in red cell uptake than the old (91 vs., 66%, respectively). However, it has been suggested (Lipschitz et al., 1986) that chronic inflammation, nutritional deficiencies, or long-term exposure to factors that suppress hematopoiesis could be reason for alterations in hematopoiesis rather than the aging process itself.

Yet a relatively recent study also found that the elderly had lower levels of iron absorption than the young (Turnlund et al.,1982a). In this study, iron was administered in conjunction with a purified formula diet, rather than in just a fasting state. The interference of dietary components would lead to a lower level of absorption than that measured in the fasting state. Seven elderly males were fed solutions enriched with a ^{58}Fe stable isotope while consuming a diet of 10 mg Fe/day. Iron absorption averaged 7.9% and approximately 0.8 mg of iron per day was absorbed. This amount is similar to an estimate for endogenous losses by the Expert Group of the World Health Organization (FAO/WHO, 1970). The authors concluded that the level given, 10 mg, would be sufficient to replace endogenous losses of this magnitude except in one individual with negative iron balance and marginal zinc nutriture. Therefore, in individuals who are unable to regulate iron absorption, 10 mg Fe/day may not be an adequate dietary level.

The only iron balance studies in *healthy* elderly were reported by Turnlund et al. in 1981. In seven healthy elderly male subjects, aged 64-74 yrs, a semi-purified diet that varied in nitrogen was fed for 42 days. Parameters of iron status were normal and some even improved, but serum ferritin was not measured. The iron intake remained at 10 mg/day throughout the study and produced negative balances in most subjects, averaging -0.44 mg/day. Inclusion of integumental losses (which were not measured) would have made the balances even more negative. Assuming body stores of 4 to 5 g of iron, iron stores would have been depleted in 10 to 15 years.

Iron balance was also measured in two older patients with pancreatic insufficiency (Wester, 1971). Iron intakes from a standard hospital diet were 4.2 and 20.4 mg/day and both produced positive balances of 2.74 and 4.75 mg, respectively.

One study (Jacobson and Webster , 1977) measured iron balance for 5 days in patients receiving iron via total parenteral administration. Three of the four subjects were elderly (66-72 yrs). In these men, a mean intravenous administration of 2.79 mg Fe/day produced mean excretory losses of 0.15 mg in the urine and 0.25 mg in the feces. Thus, the overall balance was a positive 2.26 mg/day. An intake of 0.5 mg/day was suggested as the iron requirement for patients on TPN. This value is slightly lower than the endogenous losses estimated by others (FAO/WHO, 1970; Turnlund et al., 1982a) but may reflect the needs for a hospitalized patient rather than an active healthy individual. Requirements in the sick patient may be lower than the healthy since it is well known that iron levels in serum decline with infection.

Since there are so few iron balance studies that have been conducted in the elderly, it is of interest to include the study by Hallfrisch et al. (1987). Iron balance was measured in 12 postmenopausal and 19 premenopausal women, aged 49-65, who donated replicates of their diet for 7 days and all excreta. Even though the mean dietary level of self-selected diets was the same for both the young and the old (11.8 mg/day), only the older subjects were in negative balance (-1.61 mg). When the subjects were then fed a diet high in complex carbohydrates and fiber for 91 days, iron intakes increased and balances became positive.

One factor that could increase iron requirements in the elderly is the widespread use of calcium supplements for protection against osteoporosis. In 1983, Seligman et al. found that iron supplements in prenatal vitamin/mineral supplements were less well utilized than that from just a single iron supplement. Interference from calcium was found to be partially responsible.

In 1986, Dawson-Hughes et al. measured the effect that calcium had on ^{59}Fe retention in 13 healthy, postmenopausal women, aged 59 to 70 yrs. The test of dose of 500 mg calcium as either carbonate or hydroxyapatite was given with a cereal breakfast. Hydroxapatite was chosen since it also contains phosphorus. Absorption of calcium either as the carbonate (3.2%) or the hydroxyapatite (1.7%) was significantly reduced as compared to placebo (6.3%). Thus, the presence of calcium decreased iron absorption by approximately 45%.

Monsen and Cook (1976) have also reported that a combination of calcium and phosphorus impairs the retention of nonheme iron by 53-73%. However, calcium or phosphorus alone had no effect. Snedeker et al. (1982) reported that iron retention as measured by metabolic balance was decreased, but not significantly, when a high calcium (2382 mg) and high phosphorus (2442 mg) diet was fed.

In summary, it is unclear whether or not iron absorption declines with advancing age. In women, the cessation of menses greatly reduces the excretion of iron and hence, requirements. Thus, elderly men and women have similar requirements and these may be lower than young subjects since iron stores have been reported to increase with aging. Although elderly women have lower iron stores than men, the significance of this is unclear. Judicious use of calcium supplements is recommended because of reports of interaction with inorganic iron.

CHROMIUM

Status

Measurement of chromium (Cr) status in populations has been difficult due to the inaccuracies of analytical methods. Values reported for serum chromium in 1962, for example, were 3000 times higher than that normally accepted today (Anderson et al., 1983). Thus, data from older studies must be viewed with caution unless methods of analysis and sample preparation are similar to that used today.

In the 1980's, three studies investigated dietary levels of chromium in the elderly. Of these, the highest levels, 182 µg/day, were reported by Abdulla (1986) who analyzed the duplicate 7-day diets of 37 Swedish pensioners who were 67 years old. Whether these high values are a unique situation related to Sweden or due to failure to take precautions from contamination from the blender blade during homogenization of the diet is unknown. Approximately half this level of chromium, 96 µg Cr/day, was found in the diets of 90 free-living Canadian women, aged 58-89 yr, in a study by Gibson et al. (1985). The authors commented that these chromium intakes were much higher than had been found in premenopausal women.

Much lower dietary levels were found by Bunker et al. (1984b) who reported mean chromium intakes of 20.1 and 29.8 µg/day in the diets of males and females, respectively, aged 69-85 yrs. These quantities are similar to means of 33 and 25 µg Cr/day reported in the diets of younger adult males and females, respectively, aged 25 to 65 yrs (Anderson and Kozlovsky, 1985).

Abraham et al. (1981) measured the serum chromium in 81 healthy subjects, 22 to 91 yr. The mean level of those over the age of 60 yrs was 1.9 ng/ml, compared to 1.6 ng/ml for those under this age. Although there was no significant relationship of serum chromium with increasing age in the total population, there was a significant increase in the males only. Levels in individuals with ischemic heart disease averaged 1.8 ng/ml and were not significantly different than those free of the disease.

Vir and Love (1978) studied chromium status in 196 elderly subjects residing at home or in institutions. Plasma chromium was unrelated to age except in one group of institutionalized females. In this group of subjects who received multiple vitamins, plasma chromium decreased slightly, but significantly, with advancing age.

The above reports of serum and plasma values of chromium may have little meaning since it is believed that these are not a reliable indicators of body status even though they may increase with Cr supplementation. For example, a study by Anderson et al. (1985) showed that serum Cr before and after a glucose load was not significantly different from baseline levels either during a placebo or Cr supplementation.

With the exception of lung, tissue levels of chromium have been observed to decrease with age (Schroeder et al., 1962). Furthermore, conditions associated with chromium deficiency are also associated with aging. These include impaired glucose tolerance, elevated serum cholesterol and triglycerides, increased incidence of aortic plaques and peripheral neuropathy (Anderson, 1985). Anderson commented that conditions associated with aging may more correctly be the result of long-term poor nutrition that does not become apparent until advanced age.

Yet the status of chromium in the elderly is open to question. Currently, individual response to chromium supplements is used as a diagnosis of deficiency (Anderson, 1985). Numerous studies have used supplementation of chromium or chromium-rich yeast and reported improvements in glucose tolerance and serum lipids (Anderson et al., 1985). This improvement is particularly true for elderly who are glucose-intolerant (Potter et al., 1985). In contrast, others have not found similar effects in diabetics (Sherman et al., 1968; Doisy et al., 1976). Thus, whether the glucose intolerance associated with aging (Schlenker, 1984) is a reflection of long-term inadequate chromium nutriture remains to be substantiated.

Requirement

The current estimated safe and daily dietary intake for chromium for adults is 50 to 200 μg/day (Food and Nutrition Board, 1980). This figure is derived by adding the average urinary loss of 0.8 μg (Guthrie, 1978) to a small quantity (0.2 μg) estimated for surface losses. The resultant figure, 1 μg/day, is assumed to reflect the amount of chromium that is absorbed from the diet. Combining this figure with an absorption rate of 0.5 to 0.69% (Mertz, 1969), a dietary level of 200 μg/day would meet the adult requirement.

However, the range of 50-200 μg/day is far higher than quantities found in the studies of Bunker et al. (1984b) and Anderson et al. (1985). In the first paper, balance studies were conducted on 11 healthy elderly and one subject with impaired glucose tolerance, aged 69-85 yr. The average chromium intake of 25.8 μg produced a mean positive balance of 0.2 μg/day. However, two of the subjects were in slight, and one was in severe, negative balance. But the subject with the severe negative balance had an exceptionally high fiber intake. The average absorption rate of chromium was 2.4%. The conclusion was that since the subjects were in good chromium status on this dietary level, an intake less than the current recommended level may be acceptable in well-nourished elderly. However, this intake may not be acceptable in conditions which increase requirements, such as diabetes, coronary heart disease, and situations which induce additional losses, i.e., vigorous exercise.

In the study by Offenbacher et al. (1986), urinary and fecal excreta were collected from two healthy men, ages 62 and 66, who had been fed a constant diet for 3 months. Dietary intakes of 36 µg Cr/day produced a mean positive balance of 0.4 µg/day. The positive balance on such a low dietary level of chromium led the researchers to conclude that the current ESADDI may be set too high.

Other evidence that the ESADDI may be excessive was the finding of an average urinary excretion of 0.19 µg/day when dietary intakes were 28 mg (Anderson and Kozlovsky, 1985). This urinary value is only 25% of the the level (0.8 µg) that was used in the establishment of the current ESADDI. Thus, this much lower level of urinary excretion, coupled with the much higher absorption of 2.4% reported by Bunker et al. (1984b), would suggest a lower requirement.

It should be noted that urinary excretion is no longer considered a valid indicator of the amount of dietary chromium that is absorbed or overall body status. In the past, investigators used urinary Cr excretion as a parameter of the amount absorbed and ignored fecal excretion since the amount lost in the bile was miniscule. Furthermore, it was assumed that urinary excretion remained constant regardless of dietary intake. It is now recognized that urinary excretion does change when dietary intakes are approximately 40 µg or less (Anderson and Kozlovsky, 1985).

In conclusion, further research is definitely needed to further refine chromium requirements in humans of all ages. Further quantitation of the endogenous losses via feces, as well as through integument added to urinary excretion, may result in a level that is lower than that currently suggested. A separate estimation for chromium requirements of the elderly would be premature until a consensus figure is reached for young adults.

MOLYBDENUM

Status

The dietary intakes of molybdenum (Mo) according to the Food and Drug administration's Total Diet study of 234 foods averaged 100 and 74 μg/day for males and females, respectively, ages 60-65 yrs (Pennington and Jones, 1987). Similar intakes of 99 μg/day were estimated from a study of British foods (Evans et al., 1985). Higher intakes were found in slightly older studies. These included a range of 120-240 μg/day in American foods (Tsongas et al., 1980) and 290-755 μg/day in Indian foods (Doesthale, 1980). For a review on older studies, the reader is referred to the article by Pennington and Jones (1987).

The authors are unaware of any studies that have actually measured molybdenum status in the elderly. Solomons (1986) suggested that the elderly may have less need than the young for this mineral based on its association with two enzymes. The first is xanthine oxidase, a Mo-containing enzyme that is necessary in the degradative pathway of purine metabolism. The second is Mo-containing enzyme, sulfite oxidase, which is involved in the detoxification of sulfites from amino acid metabolism. In aging, the reduction in lean body mass that occurs would lead to a diminished cellular turnover and hence, less need for metabolizing breakdown products. Also, a reduced consumption of meat would lead to fewer of these products to be metabolized. However, these possibilities are still speculative.

Requirements

The current ESADDI for molybdenum (Mo) is 150-500 μg/day (Food and Nutrition Board, 1980). This value was derived from three studies that found positive retention on diets providing 0.002 mg Mo/kg body weight or 100-150 μg/day for adults (World Health Organization, 1973). Since dietary levels less than 100 μg (48-96 μg)/day in another study (Robinson et al., 1973) produced negative balances, the lower limit was set at 150 μg as a margin of safety. An upper limit of 500 μg was established since levels of 540 μg/day were reported to increase urinary copper excretion and levels of 10-15 mg/day cause gout-like symptoms (Food and Nutrition Board, 1980).

In two older patients (52 and 62 yrs) with pancreatic insufficiency (Wester, 1971), molybdenum intakes of 250 and 930 μg/day produced negative balances of -169 and -214 μg/day. Negative balances were also seen in a study of patients on TPN (Jacobson and Webster, 1977). The three older subjects (66-72 yrs) who received solutions containing 10-11 μg/day had daily balances that ranged from -1 to -4 μg/day. The reasons for continual negative balances in these two studies are unclear.

The current recommendation for a lower limit of 150 μg/day seems appropriate if the study by Wester (1971) is ignored. Yet recent data suggest that most individuals in the United States and Britain are receiving far less and their diets may be near levels that produce negative balance. Since problems in molybdenum status have not been identified in free-living people, lower levels may be sufficient to maintain equilibrium. Future research in all population groups, as well as the elderly, is necessary before definitive recommendations can be made.

CONCLUSIONS

The precise magnitude of human requirements for many of the trace elements discussed above cannot be determined without a substantial amount of research. The current generalization that individuals in their fifties have the same metabolic requirements as those in their eighties does not seem appropriate, particularly since the elderly have increased biological variability and vast differences in health status (McGandy et al., 1986). Nutritionists must consider the effect that age-related decreased energy requirements may have on total nutrient intake, as well as changes in body composition, biochemistry, and cellular function (Freeland-Graves and Bales, this volume). The increasing number of elderly people in our society makes it imperative that health professionals more closely define parameters of optimal nutrition for this age group.

ACKNOWLEDGEMENTS

This research was supported in part by U.S. Department of Agriculture Competitive Grants Program 87-CRCR-1-2312 and University Research Institute, Biomedical Research Support Grant RR07-091-21.

REFERENCES

Aamodt RL, Rumble WF, Henkin RL (1983). Zinc absorption in humans: effects of age, sex and food. In Inglett GE (ed): "Nutritional Bioavailability of Zinc," Washington DC: American Chemical Society, ACS Symposium Series 210, pp 61-82.
Abdulla M (1986). "Inorganic Chemical Elements in Prepared Meals in Sweden," Sweden: University of Lund, pp 171-175.
Abraham AS, Sonnenblich M, Eini M (1981). Serum chromium and ageing. Gerontology 27: 326-328.
Albanese AA (1976). Nutrition and health of the elderly. Nutr News 39: 5-8.
Alhava EM, Olkkonen H, Puittinen J, Nokso-Koivisto V-M (1977). Zinc content of human cancellous bone. Acta Orthop Scand 48: 1-4.

Aggett PJ, More J, Thorn JM, Delves HT, Cornfield M, Clayton BE (1983). Evaluation of the trace metal supplements for a synthetic low lactose diet. Arch Dis Childhood 58: 433-437.
Anderson RA (1985). Chromium requirements and needs in the elderly. In Watson RR (ed): "CRC Handbook of Nutrition in the Aged," Boca Raton, Florida, CRC Press, pp 137-145.
Anderson RA, Bryden NA, Polansky MM (1985). Serum chromium of human subjects: effects of chromium supplementation and glucose. Am J Clin Nutr 41: 571-577.
Anderson RA, Kozlovsky AS (1985). Chromium intake, absorption and excretion of subjects consuming self-selected diets. Am J Clin Nutr 41: 1177-1183.
Anderson RA, Polansky MM, Bryden NA, Patterson KY, Veillon C, Glinsmann WH (1983). Effects of chromium supplementation on urinary chromium excretion of human subjects and correlation of chromium excretion with selected clinical parameters. J Nutr 113: 276-281.
Baghurst KI, Record JS (1987). The vitamin and mineral intake of a free-living young elderly Australian population in relation to total diet and supplementation practices. Hum Nutr: Appl Nutr 41A: 327-337.
Bailey LB, Wagner PA, Christakis GJ, Araujo PE, Appledorf H, Davis CG, Masteryanni J, Dinning JS (1979). Folacin and iron status and hematological findings in predominantly black elderly persons from urban low-income households. Am J Clin Nutr 32: 2346-2353.
Bales CW, Freeland-Graves JH, Lin P-H, Stone J, Dougherty V (1987). Plasma uptake of manganese: response to dose and dietary factors. In Kies C (ed): "Nutritional Bioavailability of Manganese," Washington, DC: American Chemical Society, pp 112-122.
Bales CW, Steinman LC, Freeland-Graves JH, Stone JM, Young RK (1986). The effect of age on plasma zinc uptake and taste acuity. Am J Clin Nutr 44: 664-669.
Bjorksten F, Aromaa A, Knekt P, Malinen L (1978). Serum zinc concentrations in Finns. Acta Med Scand 204: 67-74.
Bonnet JD, Hagedorn AB, Owen CA (1960). A quantitative method for measuring the gastrointestinal absorption of iron. Blood 15: 36-44.
Bunker VW, Hinks LJ, Stansfield MF, Lawson MS, Clayton BE (1987). Metabolic balance studies for zinc and copper in housebound elderly people and the relationship between zinc balance and leukocyte zinc concentrations. Am J Clin Nutr 46: 353-359.
Bunker VW, Hinks LJ, Lawson MS, Clayton BE (1984a). Assessment of zinc and copper status of healthy elderly people using metabolic balance studies and measurement of leukocyte concentrations. Am J Clin Nutr 40: 1096-1102.
Bunker VW, Lawson M, Delves HT, Clayton BE (1984b). The uptake and excretion of chromium by the elderly. Am J Clin Nutr 39: 797-802.

Bunker VW, Stansfield FM, Clayton BE (1986). The trace element and macronutrient of meals-on-wheels. Hum Nutr : Appl Nutr 40A: 323-330.

Burke DM, DeMicco FJ, Taper LJ, Ritchey SJ (1981). Copper and zinc utilization in elderly adults. J Gerontol 36: 558-563.

Casale G, Bonora C, Migliavacca A, Zurita IE, de Nicola P (1981). Serum ferritin and aging. Age and Aging 10: 119-122.

Center for Disease Control (CDC) (1972). Ten-State Nutrition Survey 1968-70. Washington DC: Health Services and Mental Health Administration. [DHEW publ no (HSM) 72-8130, 72-8133.]

Center for Food Safety and Applied Nutrition (1984). Assessment of the iron nutritional status of the U.S. population based on data collected in the second National Health and Nutrition Examination Survey, 1976-1980. Life Science Research Office, Bethesda, Maryland.

Cook JD, Finch CA, Smith NJ (1976). Evaluation of the iron status of a population. Blood 48: 449-455.

Dallman PR, Yip R, Johnson C (1984). Prevalence and causes of anemia in the United States, 1976 to 1980. Am J Clin Nutr 39: 437-445.

Dawson-Hughes B, Seligson FH, Hughes VA (1986). Effects of calcium carbonate and hydroxyapatite on zinc and iron retention in postmenopausal women. Am J Clin Nutr 44: 83-88.

Deosthale YG (1980). Molybdenum content of some common Indian foods. Ind J Nutr Dietet 18: 15-20.

DHEW (1981). Health and Nutrition Examination Survey no. 2 (HANES II). Hyattsville, MD: USPHS Division of Health Statistics.

DHEW (1979). Health and Nutrition Examination Survey no. 1 (HANES I). Hyattsville, MD: USPHS Division of Health Statistics.

Doisy RJ, Streeten DHP, Souma Ml, Kalafer ME, Rekant SL, Dalakos TG (1971). Metabolism of chromium 51 in human subjects. In Mertz W, Cornatzer WE (eds): "Newer Trace Elements in Nutrition," New York, Academic Press.

Dougherty V, Freeland-Graves J, Behmardi F, Lin P-H, Bales CW (1987). Interaction of iron (Fe) and manganese in males fed varying levels of dietary manganese (1987). Fed Proc 46: 914.

Engel RW, Price NO, Miller RF (1967). Copper, manganese, cobalt, and molybdenum balance in pre-adolescent girls. J Nutr 92: 197-204.

Engel RW, Miller RF, Price NO (1966). Metabolic patterns in preadolescent children. XIII. Zinc balance, In Prasad AS (ed): " Zinc Metabolism," Springfield, Ill., pp 326-338.

Evans WH, Read JI, Caughlin D (1985). Quantification of results for estimating elemental dietary intakes of lithium, rubidium, strontium, molybdenum, vanadium, and silver. Analyst 10: 873-877.

FAO/WHO expert group (1970). Requirements of ascorbic acid, vitamin D, vitamin B-12, folate and iron. Geneva: WHO. Technical Report Series 452.

Festa MD, Anderson HL, Dowdy RP, Ellersieck MR (1985). Effect of zinc intake on copper excretion and retention in men. Am J Clin Nutr 41: 285-292.

Finch CA, Loden B (1959). Body iron exchange in man. J Clin Inv 38: 392-396.

Finley EB, Cerklewski FL (1983). Influence of ascorbic acid supplementation on copper status in young adult men. Am J Clin Nutr 37: 553-556.

Flint DM, Wahaqvist ML, Smith TJ, Parizh AE (1981). Zinc and protein status in the elderly. J Hum Nutr 35: 287-295.

Food and Nutrition Board (1986). Recommended dietary allowances: scientific issues and process for the future. J Nutr 116:482-488.

Food and Nutrition Board (1980). Recommended Dietary Allowances, 9th Ed. Washington, DC: National Academy of Sciences.

Freedman ML, Ahronheim JC (1985). Nutritional needs of the elderly: debate and recommendations. Geriatrics 40: 45-59.

Freeland-Graves JH, Bales CW (1988). Dietary recommendations of minerals for the elderly. In Bales CW (ed): "Mineral Homeostasis in the Elderly," New York: Alan R. Liss.

Freeland-Graves JH, Behmardi F, Bales CW, Dougherty V, Lin P-H, Crosby JB, Trickett PC (1988). Metabolic balance in young men consuming diets containing five levels of dietary manganese. J Nutr 118: 764-773.

Freeland-Graves JH, Bales CW, Behmardi FB (1987). Manganese requirements in humans. In Kies C (ed): "Nutritional Bioavailability of Manganese," Washington, DC: American Chemical Society, pp 90-104.

Freeland-Graves JH, Cousins RJ, Schwatz R (1976). Relationship of mineral status and intake to periodontal disease. Am J Clin Nutr 29:754-749.

Friedman BJ, Freeland-Graves JH, Bales CW, Behmardi FB, Shorey-Kutschke R, Willis RA, Crosby JB, Trickett PC, Houston SD (1987). Manganese balance and clinical observations in young men fed a manganese deficient diet. J Nutr 117: 133-143.

Garry PJ, Goodwin JS, Hunt WC (1983). Iron status and anemia in the elderly: New findings and a review of previous studies. J Am Geriatric Soc 31: 389-399.

Garry PJ, Goodwin JS, Hunt WC, Hooper EM, Leonard AG (1982). Nutritional status in a healthy elderly population: dietary and supplemental intakes. Am J Clin Nutr 36: 319-331.

Gershoff SN, Brusis OA, Nino HV, Huber AM (1977). Studies of the elderly in Boston. 1. The effect of iron fortification on moderately anemic people. Am J Clin Nutr 30: 226-234.

Gibson RS, Mac Donald AC, Martinez OB (1985). Dietary chromium and manganese intakes of a selected sample of Canadian elderly women. Hum Nutr : Appl Nutr 39A: 43-52.

Gibson RS, Anderson BM, Sabry JH (1983). The trace metal status of a group of post-menopausal vegetarians. J Am Dietet Assoc 82: 246-250.

Gray GE, Paganini-Hill A, Ross RK (1983). Dietary intake and nutrient supplement use in a Southern California retirement community. Am J Clin Nutr 38: 122-128.

Green R, Charlton RW, Seftel H, Bothwell TH, Mayet F, Adams EB, Finch CA, Layrisse M (1968). Body iron excretion in man. A collaborative study. Am J Med 45: 336-353.

Greger JL, Baligar P, Abernathy RP, Bennett OA, Peterson TL (1978). Calcium, magnesium, phosphorus, copper and manganese balance in adolescent females. Am J Clin Nutr 31: 117-121.

Greger JL, Sciscoe BS (1977). Zinc nutriture of elderly participating in an urban feeding program. J Am Dietet Assoc 70: 37-41.

Gruden N (1977). Interrelationship of manganese and iron in rat duodenum. Nutr Rep Int 15: 577-580.

Guthrie BE, Wolf WR, Veillon C, Mertz W (1978). Chromium in urine. In Hemphill DD (ed): " Trace Substances in Environmental Health, 12," Columbia, MO: University of Missouri, pp 490-492.

Hallfrisch J, Powel A, Carafelli C, Reiser S, Prather ES (1987). Mineral balances of men and women consuming high fiber diets with complex or simple carbohydrates. J Nutr 117: 48-55.

Harman D (1965). The free radical theory of aging: effects of age on serum copper levels. J Gerontol 20: 151-153.

Hartley TF, Dawson JB, Hodgkinson A (1974). Simultaneous measurement of Na, K, Ca, Mg, Cu and Zn balances in man. Clinica Chimica Acta 52: 321-333.

Jacobs AM, Owen GM (1969). The effect of age on iron absorption. J Gerontol 24: 95-96.

Jacobson S, Wester P-O (1977). Balance study of twenty trace elements during total parenteral nutrition in man. Br J Nutr 37: 107-126.

Jeejeebhoy KN (1986). Nutritional balance studies: indicators of human requirement or adaptive mechanisms. J Nutr 116: 2061-2063.

Kelsay LJ, Prather ES (1983). Mineral balances of human subjects consuming spinach in a low-fiber diet and in a diet containing fruits and vegetables. Am J Clin Nutr 38: 12-19.

Klevay LM, Reck SJ, Jacob RA, Logan GM, Munoz JM, Sandstead HH (1980). The human requirement for copper. I. Healthy men fed conventional, American diets. Am J Clin Nutr 33: 45-50.

Kies C, Aldrich KD, Johnson JM, Creps C, Kowalski C, Wang RH (1987). Manganese availability for humans. Effect of selected dietary factors. In Kies C (ed): "Nutritional Bioavailability of Manganese," Washington, DC: American Chemical Society, pp 136-145.

Kohrs MB, Nordstrom J, Lorah PE (1980). Association of participation in a nutritional program for the elderly with nutritional status. Am J Clin Nutr 33: 2643-2656.

Kohrs MB, O'Neal R, Preston A, Eklund D, Abrahams O (1978). Nutritional status of elderly residents in Missouri. Am J Clin Nutr 31: 2186-2197.

Lin P-H, Freeland-Graves JH (1988). Effect of simultaneous ingestion of calcium and manganese in humans. In Bales C (ed): "Mineral Homeostasis in the Elderly," New York: Alan R. Liss.

Lindeman RD (1986). Mineral metabolism, aging, and the aged. In Young EA (ed): "Nutrition, Aging, and Health," New York: Alan R. Liss, pp 187-210.

Lindeman RD, Clark ML, Colmore JP (1971). Influence of age and sex on plasma and red-cell zinc concentrations. J Gerontol 26: 358-363.

Lipschitz DA (1986). Nutrition and the aging hematopoietic system. In Hutchinson ML, Munro HN (eds): "Nutrition and Aging," New York: Academic Press, pp 251-262.

Loh TT, Chang LL (1980). Hepatic iron status in Malaysians and Singaporeans. Southeast Asian J Trop Med Pub Health 11: 131-136.

Loria A, Hershko C, Konijn AM (1979). Serum ferritin in an elderly population. J Gerontol 34: 521-524.

Lynch SR, Finch CA, Monsen ER, Cook JD (1982). Iron status of eldelry Americans. Am J Clin Nutr 36: 1032-1045.

Macarthy PO, Johnson AA, Walters CS (1987). Iron nutritional status of selected elderly black persons in Washington, D.C. J Nutr Elderly 6: 3-11.

MacPhail AP, Bothwell TH, Torrance JD (1981). Iron nutrition in Indian women at different ages. S Afr Med J 59: 939-942.

Marx JJ (1979). Normal iron absorption and decreased red cell iron uptake in the aged. Blood 53: 204-211.

Masiak M, Skowron S, Owczarek H, Wodkiewicz L, Stacherzak J (1981). Serum levels of certain trace elements (Cu, Au, Mn) in healthy subjects (Part I). Acta Physiol Pol 32: 537-546.

Mason KE (1979). A conspectus of research on copper metabolism and requirements of man. J Nutr 109: 1979-2066.

McDermott SD, Kies C (1987). Manganese usage in humans as affected by use of calcium supplements. In Kies C (ed): "Nutritional Bioavailability of Manganese," Washington, DC: American Chemical Society, pp 146-151.

McLeod BE, Robinson MF (1972). Metabolic balance of manganese in young women. Br J Nutr 27: 221-227.

Mertz W (1969). Chromium occurance and function in biological systems. Physiol Rev 49: 163-239.

Monsen ER, Cook JD (1976). Food iron absorption in human subjects IV. The effects of calcium and phosphate salts on the absorption of nonheme iron. Am J Clin Nutr 29: 1142-1148.

Nordstrom JW (1982). Trace mineral nutrition in the elderly. Am J Clin Nutr 36: 788-795.

O'Dell BL, Hardwick BC, Reynolds G, Savage JE (1961). Connective tissue defect in the chick resulting from copper deficiency. Proc Soc Exp Biol Med 108: 402-405.

Offenbacher EG, Spencer H, Dowling HJ, Pi-Sunyer FX (1986). Metabolic chromium balance in man. Am J Clin Nutr 44: 77-82.

Paterson PG, Christensen DA, Robertson D (1985). Zinc levels of hospitalized elderly. J Am Dietet Assoc 85: 186-191.

Pennington JA, Jones JW (1987). Molybdenum, nickle, cobalt, vanadium, and strontium in total diets. J Am Dietet Assoc 87: 1644-1650.

Pennington JA, Young BE, Wilson DB, Johnson RD, Vanderveen JE (1986). Mineral content of foods and total diets: The selected minerals in foods survey, 1982 to 1984. J Am Dietet Assoc 86: 876-891.

Petering HG, Yeager DW, Witherup SO (1971). Trace metal content of hair I. Zinc and copper content of human hair in relation to age and sex. Arch Environ Health 23: 202-207.

Pilch SM, Senti FR (1984). Assessment of the zinc nutritional status of the US population based on data collected in HANES II survey. 1976-1980. Rockville, MD: Fed Am Soc Exp Biol (Life Science Research Office).

Potter JF, Levin P, Anderson RA, Freiberg JM, Andres R, Elahi D (1985). Glucose metabolism in glucose-intolerant older people during chromium supplementation. Metabolism 34: 199-204.

Price NO, Bunce GE, Engel RW. (1970). Copper, manganese, and zinc balance in preadolescent girls. Am J Clin Nutr 23: 258-260.

Reiser S, Ferretti RJ, Fields M, Smith JC (1983). Role of dietary fructose in the enhancement of mortality and biochemical changes associated with copper deficiency in rats. Am J Clin Nutr 38: 214-222.

Robinson MF, McKenzie JM, Thomson CD, van Rij AL (1973). Metabolic balance of zinc, copper, cadmium, iron, molybdenum and selenium in young New Zealand women. Br J Nutr 30: 195-205.

Sandstead HH (1982a). Copper bioavailability and requirements. Am J Clin Nutr 35: 809-814.

Sandstead HH, Henriksen LK, Greger JL, Prasad AS, Good RA (1982b). Zinc nutriture in the elderly in relation to taste acuity, immune response, and wound healing. Am J Clin Nutr 36: 1046-1059.

Schlenker, E(1984). Nutrition in Aging. St. Louis, Missouri: Times Mirror/Mosby p. 116.

Schroeder HA, Balassa JJ, Tipton IH (1962). Abnormal trace metals in man - chromium. J Chron Dis 15: 941-964.

Schroeder HA, Nason AP, Tipton IH, Balassa JJ (1966). Essential trace elements in man : copper. J Chron Dis 19: 1007-1021.

Schroeder HA, Nason AP, Tipton IH, Balassa JJ (1967). Essential trace metals in man : zinc. Relation to environmental cadmium. J Chron Dis 20: 179-210.

Schor RA, Prussin SG, Jewett DC, Kudowieg JJ, Bhatnagar RS (1973). Trace levels of manganese, copper, and zinc in rib cartilage as related to age in humans and animals, both normal and dwarfed. Clin Orthop 93: 346-355

Schwartz R, Apgar BJ, Wien E M (1986). Apparent absorption and retention of Ca, Cu, Mg, Mn, and Zn from a diet containing bran. Am J Clin Nutr 43:444-455.

Seligman PA, Caskey JH, Frazier JL, Zucker RM, Podell R, Allen RH (1983). Measurements of iron absorption from prenatal multivitamin-mineral supplements. Obstet Gynecol 61: 356-362.

Sherman L, Glennon JA, Brech WJ (1968). Failure of trivalent chromium to improve hyperglycemia in diabetes mellitus. Metabolism 17: 439-442.

Shields GS, Coulson WF, Kimball DA, Carnes WH, Cartwright GE, Wintrobe MM (1962). Studies on copper metabolism. XXXII, Cardiovascular lesions in copper-deficient swine. Am J Pathol 41: 603-621.

Shike M, Roulet M, Kurian R, Whitwell J, Stewart S, Jeejeebhoy KN (1981). Copper metabolism and requirements in total parenteral nutrition. Gastroenter 81: 290-297.

Smith JC, Morris ER, Ellis R (1983). Zinc: Requirements, bioavailability and recommended dietary allowance. In "Zinc Deficiency in Human Subjects," New York: Alan R Liss, Inc., pp 147-169.

Snedeker SM, Smith SA, Greger JL (1982). Effect of dietary calcium and phosphorous levels on the utilization of iron, copper, and zinc by adult males. J Nutr 112: 136-143.

Solomons N (1986a). Trace elements in nutrition of the elderly 1. Established RDAs for iron, zinc, and iodine. Postgrad Med 79: 231-242.

Solomons N (1986b). Trace elements in nutrition of the elderly 2. SADDIs for copper, manganese, selenium, chromium, molybdenum, and fluoride. Postgrad Med 79: 251-263.

Spencer HD, Osis LK, Noris C (1976). Intake, excretion, and retention of zinc in man. In Prasad AS (ed): " Trace Elements in Human Health and Disease," New York: Academic Press, pp 345-361.

Strause LG, Hegenauer J, Saltman P, Cone R, Resnick D (1986). Effects of long-term dietary manganese and copper deficiency on rat skeleton. J Nutr. 116:135-141.

Strause L, Saltman P (1987). Role of manganese in bone metabolism. In Kies C (ed): "Nutritional Bioavailability of Manganese," Washington DC: American Chemical Society, pp 45-55.

Sullivan JF, Blotcky AJ, Jetton MM, Hahn HK, Burch RE. (1979). Serum levels of selenium, calcium, copper, magnesium, manganese and zinc in various human diseases. J Nutr 109: 1432-1437.

Taper TJ, Hinners Ml, Ritchey SJ (1980). Effects of zinc intake on copper balance in adult females. Am J Clin Nutr 33: 1077-1082.

Taylor GO, Williams AO (1974). Lipid and trace metal content in coronary arteries of Nigerian Africans. Exp Mol Path 21: 371-380.

Truswell AS (1986). New and recent recommended dietary intakes and dietary guidelines : a workshop report. In Taylor TG, Jenkins NK (eds): "Proceedings of the XIII International Congress of Nutrition," London: John Libbey, pp 957-960.

Truswell AS (1983). Recommended dietary intakes around the world - Introduction. Nutr Abs Rev Clin Nutr - Series A 53: 940-1015.

Tsongas TA, Meglen RR, Walravens PA, Chappell WR (1980). Molybdenum in the diet: an estimate of average daily intake in the United States. Am J Clin Nutr 33: 1103-1107.

Turnlund JR, Durkin N, Costa F, Margen S (1986). Stable isotope studies of zinc absoption and retention in young and elderly men. J Nutr 116: 1239-1247.

Turnlund JR, Michel MC, Keyes WR, King JC, Margen S (1982a). Use of enriched stable isotopes to determine zinc and iron absorption in elderly men. Am J Clin Nutr 35: 1033-1040.

Turnlund JR, Michel MC, Keyes WR, Schutz Y, Margen S (1982b). Copper absorption in elderly men determined by using stable ^{65}Cu. Am J Clin Nutr 36: 587-591.

Turnlund J, Costa F, Margen S (1981). Zinc, copper, and iron balance in elderly men. Am J Clin Nutr 34: 2641-2647.

Valberg LS, Sorbier J, Ludwig J, Pelletier O (1976). Serum ferritin and the iron status of Canadians. Canad Med Assoc J 114: 417-421.

Vir SC, Love AHG (1978). Chromium status of the aged. Int J Vitam Nutr Res 48: 402-404.

Vir SC, Love AHG (1979). Zinc and copper status of the elderly. Am J Clin Nutr 32: 1472-1476.

Wagner PA, Bailey LB, Krista ML, Jernigan JA, Robinson JD, Cerda JJ (1981). Comparison of zinc and folacin status in elderly women from differing socioeconomic backgrounds. Nutr Res 1: 565-569.

Wagner PA, Krista ML, Bailey LB, Christakis GJ, Jernigan JA, Araujo PR, Appledorf H, Davis CG, Denning JS (1980). Zinc status of elderly black Americans from urban low-income households. Am J Clin Nutr 33: 1771-1777.

Wester PO (1971). Trace element balances in two cases of pancreatic insufficiency. Acta Med Scand 190: 155-161.

Wolman SL, Anderson GH, Marliss EB, Jeejeebhoy KN(1979). Zinc in total parenteral nutrition: requirements and metabolic effects. Gastroenterology 76: 458-467.

World Health Organization (1973). Zinc. WHO Tech Rep Ser 532: 9-16.

Yunice AA, Lindeman RD, Czerwinski AW, Clark M (1974). Influence of age and sex on serum copper and ceruloplasmin levels. J Gerontol 29: 277-281.

Mineral Homeostasis in the Elderly, pages 171–199
© *1989 Alan R. Liss, Inc.*

POTENTIAL FOR TRACE MINERAL DEFICIENCIES AND TOXICITIES IN
THE ELDERLY

Janet L. Greger, Ph.D.

Department of Nutritional Sciences
University of Wisconsin
Madison, WI 53706

More than thirteen elements are currently believed to be
required by mammals in trace amounts. Many other elements
are found in mammalian tissues but have no known function.
Unfortunately, limited data are available on the utilization
of most of these trace elements by human subjects,
especially by elderly subjects. Thus this discussion will
be focused on the potential for deficiencies of zinc and
copper and for toxicity from aluminum among the elderly.

ZINC

Zinc Intake of the Elderly

At least seventeen different groups of investigators have
reported the zinc intakes of elderly individuals in North
America, Europe and Australia during the last fifteen
years. The results of these small-scale surveys have been
fairly consistent. Investigators have generally observed
that the average elderly individual consumed 7 to 11 mg.
zinc daily (Abdulla et al., 1977; Greger and Siscoe, 1977;
Greger, 1977; Stiedemann and Harrill, 1980; Flint et al.,
1981; Anderson et al., 1981; Sempos et al. 1982; Wagner et
al., 1983; Hutton and Hayes-Davis, 1983; Betts and Vivian,
1984; Brooks and Cummings, 1984; Fosmire et al., 1984;
Bunker et al., 1984; McGandy et al., 1986; Bogden et al.,
1987; Bunker et al., 1987; Sahyoun et al., 1988). That
means that the average elderly individual in these surveys
consumed 47 to 73% of the amount of zinc suggested in the

Recommended Dietary Allowances (RDA) (Food and Nutrition Board, 1980).

Although a large number of elderly individuals in several of these surveys used nutrient supplements, the supplements used did not generally increase the zinc intake of subjects (Greger, 1977; Anderson et al., 1981; McGandy et al., 1986; Sahyoun et al., 1988) For example, McGandy et al. (1986) observed that 60% and 55% of their subjects older than 80 years of age consumed less than two-thirds of the RDA for zinc from diet and from diet and supplements, respectively.

Several factors were identified in these surveys that can be used to predict which elderly are apt to have low zinc intakes. Elderly women usually consumed less zinc than elderly men. On average, those elderly individuals who resided in an institution or who were homebound consumed less zinc than free-living subjects in the same locale (Greger and Sciscoe, 1977; Greger, 1977; Flint et al., 1981; Bunker et al., 1984; Bunker et al., 1987).

Unfortunately zinc intakes have not been reported for elderly subjects in any large nationwide survey. However, useful information pertinent to the topic of zinc intake of the elderly can be gleaned from a 1977 food consumption survey by the U.S. Department of Agriculture (USDA) (Science and Education Administration, 1980). In that survey, the average man and woman older than 75 years of age consumed 26% and 15%, respectively, less energy daily than the average young (23-34 years of age) man and woman.

Analysis of data from that survey demonstrated that not only did the elderly consume less food than younger adults, they also made different food choices. The average man and woman over 75 years of age consumed 31% and 17% respectively, less meat, fish, and poultry than young (23-35 years of age) adults. This change in types of foods consumed would affect zinc intakes because meat, fish and poultry are the primary sources of zinc in the diets of Americans (Welsh and Marston, 1982).

It is likely that the majority of the elderly in the United States, particularly women and those individuals older than 75 years, consume less than two-thirds of the RDA for zinc. This conclusion does not mean that the majority of elderly Americans are consuming inadequate amounts of zinc to meet their needs. It does suggest that a large percentage of the elderly may be at risk of consuming inadequate amounts of zinc. Whether these individuals would benefit from additional zinc depends on a variety of factors.

Factors that Affect Zinc Requirements of the Elderly

The zinc requirements of humans of any age are not well-defined (Hambidge et al., 1986). Usually the average elderly subject in metabolic studies achieved balance (i.e. intake > fecal and urinary losses) in regard to zinc when they consumed 8 to 15 mg zinc daily (Burke et al., 1981; Turnlund et al., 1981; Spencer et al., 1982; Bunker et al., 1982; Bunker et al., 1984; Turnlund et al., 1986; Bunker et al., 1987). The exact level at which balance was achieved in these studies was dependent on a number of factors.

Turnlund et al. (1986) observed that elderly men absorbed zinc less efficiently than young men fed similar diets (18% vs 32% absorption). However, the elderly men excreted less endogenous zinc from the gut than the young men. Thus the two age groups did not differ in regard to fecal zinc losses or zinc balance. These results could be interpreted in two ways: 1) The need for dietary zinc, as evidenced by decreased endogenous zinc loss, declined with age. Thus the efficiency of zinc absorption declined. 2) The efficiency of zinc absorption declined with age. To compensate the elderly excreted less endogenous zinc. If the latter mechanism did not adjust sufficiently, zinc requirements were increased.

Effect of disease. The elderly individuals, who participated in most of the metabolic studies cited, were healthy. Many elderly individuals have disease states or use medication that are known to impair the utilization of zinc (Sandstead et al., 1982). Thus their zinc requirements are accordingly elevated.

Urinary losses of zinc are generally small in normal subjects; they usually account for less than 7% of dietary intake (Hambidge et al., 1986). However, in several pathological conditions (e.g. skeletal injuries, surgery and burns) urinary losses of zinc are large enough to be of practical significance and serum zinc levels fall (Cohen et al., 1973; Askari et al., 1979). Conditions that cause muscle wasting (Fell et al., 1973; Henkin et al., 1975) and alcohol-induced cirrhosis of the liver (Prosad, 1979) have also been found to increase urinary zinc losses significantly. Part of the increased urinary zinc losses observed in several of these conditions is attributable to the muscle and bone atrophy that occurs during complete bed rest (Krebs et al., 1988).

Effect of medications. Diuretics, including thiazides, chlorthalidone and furosemide, increase urinary excretion of zinc (Roe, 1976), Wester (1980) noted that although serum zinc levels of patients taking diuretics remained in the normal range, tissue levels of zinc were depressed in patients who received diuretic therapy for six months or longer.

Many elderly individuals consume fiber and calcium supplements daily. It is well documented that the consumption of large quantities of fiber, especially if phytate is present, will depress zinc absorption (Sandstead, 1982a; Solomons, 1982). Moreover, supplementation of diets that contain high levels of phytate with calcium has been found to depress zinc absorption even more (Fordyce et al., 1987). However, Sandström et al. (1983) observed no change in serum zinc levels among elderly patients when bran was added to their diets.

Bioavailability of dietary zinc. A variety of dietary components have been found to depress zinc absorption. These include fiber (Sandstead, 1982a; Solomons, 1982), phytate (Solomons, 1982; Greger, 1982), calcium in the presence of high levels of phosphorus or phytate (Greger, 1982; Fordyce et al., 1987), and tin (Johnson et al., 1982). The last factor may be more important among the elderly than in the general population because of the popularity of canned foods among the elderly, particularly edentulous elderly. Two groups of investigators have observed that elevation of dietary protein levels improved zinc absorption (Greger and Snedeker, 1980; Spencer et al., 1982) but this effect was not observed by another group (Turnlund et al., 1981). All of these factors are more apt to affect significantly zinc utilization of individuals whose intakes of zinc are marginal.

Clinical Evaluation of Nutritional Status in Regard to Zinc

Circulating zinc levels. There is no universally accepted way to monitor nutritional status of patients in regard to zinc. Plasma and serum zinc levels are the most commonly used indicators of nutritional status in regard to zinc. Although there has been considerable debate over the relative merits of serum versus plasma zinc levels, a Life Sciences Research Office (1984) panel judged them to be equivalent.

There are a number of problems involved with using circulating zinc levels as an index of nutritional status. Circulating levels of zinc have been found to be depressed in patients with acute infections, traumatic injuries, hepatic encephalopathy, or neoplastic disease (Cohen et al., 1973; Henkin et al., 1975; Sullivan et al, 1979; Reding et al., 1984). The changes may reflect losses of zinc from the individuals' total body stores of zinc and/or changes in the distribution of zinc among tissues. Diurnal variations, probably related to the ingestion of food, have also been noted in circulating zinc levels (Life Science Research Office, 1984).

Given these confounding factors, it is not surprising that investigators have used different standards for defining low serum or plasma zinc levels in various studies (Table 1). Hence, investigators have reported the incidence of poor nutritional status in regard to zinc, as determined by plasma or serum zinc levels, to range from 2 to 61% of the elderly participants in various surveys (Table 1).

Lindeman et al. (1971) noted that elderly subjects tended to have lower plasma zinc levels than younger subjects; Chooi et al. (1976) observed plasma zinc levels were decreased among healthy adults older than 50 years of age. However, other investigators have not been able to confirm these observations in small surveys (Vir and Love, 1979; Wagner et al., 1980; Flint et al., 1981). Careful analysis of the data collected in the HANES-II survey suggested that serum zinc levels tended to be lower among individuals aged 65-74 years than among young adults (Life Science Research Office, 1984). The difference was more obvious among males than females.

TABLE 1: Zinc levels in plasma and serum samples from elderly individuals

Age of subjects	No. of subjects	Mean plasma or serum zinc levels (µg/dl)	% of subjects with low zinc levels	Reference
34-82	80	92	NR[a]	Husain and Bessent, 1974
41-91	187	110	10[b]	Fisher et al., 1978
65-95	146	79	2[c]	Vir and Love, 1979
60-87	91	93	7[d]	Wagner et al., 1980
67-96	36	78	61[e]	Stiedemann and Harrill, 1980
60-99	90	91	26[e]	Flint et al., 1981
53	47	99	15[d]	Anderson et al., 1981
60-97	89	92	6[d]	Wagner et al., 1983
65-74(male)	982	86	3[f]	Life Science Research Office, 1984
65-74(female)	1153	84	3[f]	Life Science Research Office, 1984
62-84	48	93	NR[a]	Brooks and Cummings, 1984
65-90	44	105	5[d]	Fosmire et al., 1984
63-104	91	72	67[g]	Paterson et al., 1985
60-89	95	85	15[d]	Bogden et al., 1987
>60(male)	257	97	5[d]	Sahyoun et al., 1988

[a] Not reported.
[b] <81 µg/dl defined as low level.
[c] <50 µg/dl defined as low level.
[d] <70 µg/dl defined as low level.
[e] <80 µg/dl defined as low level.
[f] Variable definition of low: <70µ/dl on samples collected in a.m. from fasted subjects;
    <65µ/dl on samples collected in a.m. from non-fasted subjects; <60µ/dl on samples
    collected in p.m. from non-fasted subjects.
[g] <79 µg/dl defined as low level.

<u>Hair zinc levels</u>. Several investigators have used concentrations of zinc in hair samples from patients as an indication of nutritional status in regard to zinc. The noninvasive nature of this analysis has made it appealing. However, the levels of zinc in hair samples have not always been found to be related to the zinc intakes of animals and humans (Hambidge et al., 1986; Klevay et al., 1987). Contamination of samples was probably a problem in some cases.

The average levels of zinc reported in hair samples from elderly subjects have ranged from 140–222 µg Zn/g (Greger and Sciscoe, 1977; Greger, 1977; Vir and Love, 1979; Wagner et al., 1980; Wagner et al., 1981; Anderson et al., 1981; Wagner et al., 1983; Hutton and Hayes–Davis, 1983; Brooks and Cummings, 1984; Fosmire et al., 1984; Bogden et al., 1987). Generally the average concentrations of zinc in the hair samples from elderly subjects has been found to be less than those from young adults and adolescents by investigators who have studied several groups (Greger and Sciscoe, 1977; Greger, 1977; Wagner et al., 1981; Wagner et al., 1983). Hair samples from only a few elderly subjects (0–8%) contained less than 70 µg zinc/g hair, a concentration that has often been used to define low hair zinc levels.

<u>Other biochemical indices of zinc status.</u> Several investigators have attempted to utilize leukocyte zinc levels (Bunker et al., 1984; Bogden et al., 1987; Bunker et al., 1987) and serum alkaline phosphatase levels (Paterson et al., 1985; Bogden et al., 1987) as measures of nutritional status in regard to zinc among the elderly. Generally these variables were not found to be correlated to plasma zinc concentrations, zinc intakes, or metabolically determined zinc balances. However, Bunker et al. (1984, 1987) observed a highly significant correlation between zinc balance and leukocyte zinc levels among homebound elderly subjects, but not among healthy elderly subjects. Several of these homebound subjects had particularly low zinc intakes (<5 mg zinc daily).

Clinical Evidence of Zinc Deficiency Among the Elderly

The limited usefulness of all of these measures in defining marginal nutritional status in regard to zinc have encouraged the development of functional tests. Moreover,

some of the symptoms of zinc deficiency, (i.e. slow wound
healing, anorexia, dermatitis, depressed taste acuity,
impaired immune function) resemble common problems observed
among the elderly.

Taste acuity. A number of investigators have noted that
elderly subjects had higher taste detection levels for
sodium chloride and sucrose than young adults using
standardized tests for taste acuity (Cooper et al., 1959;
Greger and Sciscoe, 1977; Greger, 1977; Wagner et al., 1981;
Hutton and Hayes-Davis, 1983; Bales et al., 1986). (High
taste detection levels indicate poor taste acuity.)
However, investigators have been unable to find correlations
between the nutritional status of the elderly in regard to
zinc and taste acuity.

Two double blind zinc supplementation studies have also
been conducted to examine the relationship between
nutritional status in regard to zinc and taste acuity.
Greger and Geissler (1978) in a double blind study
administered either 15 gm zinc daily or placebo tablets to
49 elderly individuals for 95 days. No significant changes
were observed in the taste acuity of subjects, although hair
zinc levels increased in the individuals receiving the zinc
supplements. Seligson (1980) confirmed these observations
in another study with 113 elderly individuals.

Although zinc deficiency may not be related to the
depressed taste acuity observed among the aged, Morley
(1986) has suggested that marginal nutritional status in
regard to zinc may be related to the anorexia that is often
observed among infirm individuals. The effect of improved
zinc status on the appetite of the elderly, particularly the
infirm, has not been evaluated.

Wound healing. Zinc is essential for wound healing
(Hambidge et al., 1986). However, it is not clear that the
nutritional status of most elderly individuals in regard to
zinc is a significant factor affecting wound healing.

In two double blind therapeutic trials investigators
reported that leg ulcers healed more rapidly among subjects
given zinc supplements (Halböök and Lanner, 1972; Haeger et
al., 1974). However, in one study the zinc status of the
subjects was not evaluated. In the other study, the
investigators found that only those subjects with serum zinc

levels of less than 110 µg/100 ml responded to large zinc
supplements (600 mg zinc sulfate daily) (Halböök and Lanner,
1972).

Weismann et al. (1978) found 26 elderly individuals with
"skin manifestations suggestive of chronic zinc deficiency"
in an institution for the elderly. Ten of the subjects had
subnormal (<70 µg/dl) plasma zinc levels; they were
treated for four weeks with zinc sulfate tablets (0.6
g/day). Although the plasma zinc levels of subjects rose,
there were no improvements in the skin conditions of the
patients.

Immune function. Antibody-mediated responses to both T
cell-dependent and T cell-independent antigens, natural
killer cell activity, and delayed-type hypersensitivity are
all reduced during zinc deficiency (Fraker et al, 1986).
Several groups of investigators have hypothesized that poor
nutritional status in regard to zinc might be related to the
impaired immune function sometimes observed among the
elderly (Stiedemann and Harrill, 1980; Wagner et al., 1983;
Prasad, 1986; Ventura et al., 1986; Bogden et al., 1987).

The data from each of these studies are difficult to
interpret because of methodological limitations. Duchateau
and his associates (1981) administered 100 mg zinc daily to
15 elderly subjects for one month. The group given the zinc
supplements exhibited significant improvements in regard to
several immunological variables. No attempt was made to
monitor circulating zinc levels.

Wagner et al. (1983) found that 22% of the 173 elderly
subjects that they surveyed were nonresponsive to four
standard antigens. Five months after the original survey,
five of these subjects were restudied and found to still be
anergic. After four weeks of treatment with oral doses of
55 mg zinc daily, these five elderly subjects developed
positive responses to skin tests. Their initial serum zinc
levels ranged from 64 to 75 µg/dl; their serum zinc levels
after the treatment ranged from 89 to 128 µg/dl.

Ventura et al. (1986) demonstrated that the addition of
zinc to in vitro systems increased in the natural killer
activity of lymphocytes from elderly subjects to the level
of activity in lymphocytes from young subjects.

Recently Bogden et al. (1987) reported a high incidence of anergia to a panel of seven skin test antigens among elderly subjects. Plasma zinc concentrations were significantly higher among subjects who responded to two or more skin test antigens than among those who did not. However, zinc levels in mononuclear cells, leukocytes and platelets did not differ between responders and nonresponders to skin tests.

The effects of zinc supplements on the immunocompetence of both infirm and healthy elderly individuals need to be evaluated with double blind trials. Both nutritional and pharmacological doses of zinc should be evaluated. The latter studies are important in light of two reports: Chandra (1984) has observed that ingestion of excess zinc depressed immune function in young men, And Rao (1982) has observed that the addition of zinc to in vitro systems enhanced concanavalin A-induced capping of lymphocytes from young subjects but suppressed this activity in lymphocytes from elderly subjects.

Several investigators have noted low circulating zinc levels among individuals with malignancies (Prasad, 1979; Sullivan et al., 1979; Murphy et al., 1985). This may reflect the effect of the tumors or protective adaptive responses by the hosts. Several investigators have observed that growth of tumors was inhibited in zinc-depleted animals (Minkel et al, 1979; Mills et al., 1984). The significance of low tissue zinc levels among elderly individuals need to be evaluated not only in regard to immunocompetence but also in regard to the promotion of malignancies.

In general, clinical evidence of impaired nutritional status in regard to zinc among the elderly is limited. More studies are needed before scientists can estimate the true significance of the apparently low dietary intakes of zinc by the elderly and their sometimes low circulating levels of zinc.

COPPER

Copper Intake of the Elderly

The estimated safe and adequate daily dietary intake (SAI) for copper suggested by the Food and Nutrition Board (1980) is 2 to 3 mg copper daily. During the last fifteen years, investigators have repeatedly shown that average "Western style" diets contained 1.0 to 1.5 mg copper daily (Klevay et al., 1979; Pennington et al., 1986).

The few investigators who have attempted to estimate the copper intakes of elderly subjects have concluded that the elderly consume similar levels of copper as young adults (Pennington et al., 1986; Thomas et al., 1986). Those individuals, who have reduced intakes of energy, especially the infirm elderly, are apt to have reduced intakes of copper. The distribution of copper in foodstuffs is such that food selection patterns of the elderly are not apt to adversely affect their copper intakes (Greger, 1986).

It is difficult to evaluate the significance of the observation that probably most elderly individuals consume approximately 50% of the SAI for copper. Food composition tables list the copper content of a limited number of foods. A variety of factors, including soil conditions and varieties of plants, can alter the copper content of food items by several fold (Schletwein-Gsell and Mommsen-Straub, 1971; Pennington and Calloway, 1973).

Factors that Affect Copper Metabolism

Scientists at the USDA laboratory at Grand Forks have found that young men must consume about 1.3 mg copper in a mixed diet in order to compensate for fecal and urinary losses (Sandstead et al., 1978; Klevay et al., 1980). Subjects were found to lose an additional 0.25 mg copper per day in sweat. Thus the requirement for copper was estimated to be 1.55 mg copper daily.

The minimum amount of dietary copper required by elderly adults is probably similar to that required by young adults. Turnlund et al. (1984) found no difference in the apparent absorption of copper by elderly and young adults. Generally, elderly subjects participating in balance studies have tended to be in positive balance in regard to copper when they consumed ≥ 2.0 mg copper daily (Burke et al., 1981; Turnlund et al., 1982) and have tended to be negative balance in regard to copper when they consumed <1.3 mg copper daily (Bunker et al 1984; Bunker et al., 1987).

A variety of dietary factors can affect copper utilization
(Sandstead, 1982b). The addition of phytate and fiber to
human diets tends to depress copper absorption, but the
addition of protein to human diet tends to improve copper
absorption (Greger and Snedeker, 1980; Turnlund et al.,
1981; Sandstead, 1982b). The ingestion of fructose rather
than starch has been associated with depressed cuprozinc
superoxide dismutase activity in red blood cells of human
subjects fed 1.03 mg copper daily also (Reiser et al.,
1985). Ingestion of ascorbic acid supplements has also been
found to depress serum ceruloplasmin levels in subjects
(Finley and Cerklewski, 1983). Moreover, copper absorption
is sensitive to fairly small increments in zinc intake
(Greger et al., 1978; Sandstead, 1982b).

Disease states and medications that alter copper
metabolism. The metabolism of copper is affected by a
variety of disease states and medications. Patients and
animal models with cancer, rheumatoid arthritis, emphysema,
congestive heart failure, infections, psychoses or biliary
cirrhosis have all been found to have elevated circulating
levels of copper (Sullivan et al., 1979; Askari et al.,
1980; Youssef et al., 1983; Klevay, 1984; Murphy et al.,
1985) and often have been reported to have elevated plasma
ceruloplasmin levels (Deering et al., 1977; Karp et al.,
1986; Murphy et al., 1985).

Askari et al. (1985) even suggested that serum copper
levels might be clinically useful in the evaluation of the
efficacy of treatment among cancer patients. The mechanisms
causing the elevation of plasma copper levels in cancer
patients are generally unknown. Cohen et al. (1979)
observed that rats bearing tumors absorbed copper more
efficiently than control rats. Karp et al. (1986) noted
slower body turnover of copper in tumor-bearing rats.
However, Garofalo et al. (1980) questioned whether some of
the elevations in serum copper levels ascribed to the
effects of malignancies should be ascribed to age.

Serum levels of copper are also elevated in patients for
at least six days after surgery (Gregoriadis et al., 1982).
Therapy with estrogens and diuretics have also been found to
elevate circulating levels of copper (Sempos et al., 1983;
Karp, 1986).

Clinical Evaluation of Nutritional Status in Regard to Copper

The variables most often used to monitor nutritional status in regard to copper have been plasma and serum levels of copper and ceruloplasmin. Hypocupremia is an early and fairly consistent manifestation of experimental copper deficiency in animals (Underwood, 1977). However, as already noted, circulating levels of copper and ceruloplasmin are affected by a variety of disease states and medications. Moreover, females tend to have somewhat higher circulating levels of copper and ceruloplasmin than males (Denko and Gabriel, 1981). Diurnal variations in plasma copper have also been noted (Lifschitz and Henkin, 1971).

In small surveys, investigators found no evidence of low plasma or serum copper or ceruloplasmin levels among elderly subjects (Vir and Love, 1979; Garofalo et al., 1980; Denko and Gabriel, 1981; Schreurs et al., 1982; Sempos et al., 1983). This may reflect an increased incidence of health problems, that elevated plasma copper and ceruloplasmin levels, among the elderly or a natural increase in plasma copper levels with age. Garofalo et al. (1980) found that 60 females (ages 20 to 45 years of age) had significantly lower levels of copper in their serum than 26 older females (67 to 98 years of age). Sempos et al. (1983) observed a weak correlation between age and serum copper levels among 137 women (35 to 67 years of age). Schreurs et al. (1982) observed an elevation in serum copper levels among men older than 60 years but not among women. Denko and Gabriel (1981) observed both men and women older than 55 years of age have elevated levels of ceruloplasmin in their serum. But Vir and Love (1979) noted no correlation between plasma copper levels and age among 53 elderly subjects.

Serum copper levels were monitored in more than 14,000 individuals participating in the Second Health and Nutrition Examination Survey (HANES II) (Fulwood et al., 1982). In the survey gender, economic status and race all were found to significantly affect serum copper levels. Age (at least among adults) was not found to significantly serum copper levels of participants in this large survey. Only 1.6% and 0.3% of the elderly men and elderly women (65–74 years of age), respectively, participating in HANES II survey had plasma copper levels below <80 µg/dl.

Thus the incidence of poor nutritional status in regard to copper among the elderly appears to be minimal. Of course, disease states that elevate circulating copper levels are confounding factors. Moreover, better methods of assessing nutritional status in regard to copper need to be developed. Hair copper levels are not a useful index of nutritional status in regard to copper (Klevay et al., 1987). Cytosolic superoxide dismutase (Cu-Zn SOD) appears to be the most promising assay (Uaoy et al., 1985).

Significance of Alterations in Copper Metabolism Among the Elderly

Several investigators, notably Klevay (1984), have demonstrated that the long term consumption of marginally adequate levels (i.e. <1.0 mg daily) of copper or the consumption of factors that suppress utilization of copper produced hypercholesterolemia in animal models (Petering et al., 1977; Lei, 1978; Law and Klevay, 1981; Harvey and Allen, 1981; Milne et al., 1981; Lei, 1983; Klevay, 1984; Croswell and Lei, 1985; Lefevre et al., 1986). The mechanism(s) by which copper deficiency induced changes in cholesterol metabolism is not clear. Cholesterol degration appeared to be impaired in copper deficient rats (Lei, 1978; Lei, 1983)., Lefevre et al. (1986) observed that hepatic membranes of copper deficient rats bound fewer lipoproteins than those of controls. Thus there were marked increases in apo E-rich HDL levels.

The significance of low copper intakes by young, middle-aged and elderly individuals in the etiology of ischemic heart disease has not been fully assessed. It deserves further study.

In general, it appears that many Americans consume less than recommended levels of copper. The long term consequences of consumption of marginally adequate levels of copper are not clear. Furthermore, the sensitivity of plasma copper and ceruloplasmin levels to a variety of disease states makes it difficult to monitor the nutritional status in regard to copper of any group of individuals, especially the elderly.

ALUMINUM

Aluminum is not believed to be an essential element; it is thought to exert toxic affects when it accumulates in tissues (Greger, 1987). Thus many clinicians are interested in the assessing exposure to aluminum and in monitoring tissue accumulation of aluminum.

Aluminum Intake

Only a limited amount of data are available on the aluminum content of foodstuffs. Moreover, estimates of the aluminum content of biological samples should be viewed with skepticism. During the last 20 years, estimates of the amount of aluminum in serum samples have decreased 50-fold because of improvements in methodology (Versieck and Cornelis, 1980).

Despite these limitations, it appears that the average adult consuming a "Western-style" diet consumes 20-40 mg aluminum daily in food and beverages (Greger, 1985). A few consume as little as 2 mg aluminum daily; a few consume more than 100 mg aluminum daily. The sources of dietary aluminum are natural sources, food additives and contamination from containers and utensils. Food additives are the primary source of dietary aluminum for most Americans.

The quantities of aluminum consumed in food and beverages are small compared to the amounts of aluminum that can be ingested in pharmaceutical products, such as antacids, buffered analgesics, antidiarrheals and certain antiulcer drugs (Lione, 1985). Lione (1985) estimated that 800-5000 mg aluminum and 126-728 mg aluminum were possible daily doses of aluminum in antacids and buffered analgesics, respectively.

Clinical Consequences of Excess Exposure to Aluminum

Aluminum intoxication has been reported among uremic patients undergoing dialysis with aluminum-contaminated dialysate fluids and among patients receiving prolonged intravenous infusions, especially with aluminum contaminated albumin (King et al., 1981; Alfrey, 1986). The clinical picture generally includes osteodystrophy, encephalopathy, and/or anemia. The symptoms of the osteodystrophy often include increased bone pain and fractures and a bone histology that is consistent with osteomalacia with aluminum accumulation in bone. The symptoms of the encephalopathy include dementia, speech difficulties, motor abnormalities and/or abnormal electroencephalograms. On autopsy, the tissues of patients with dialysis encephalopathy (dialysis dementia) have been found to contain greatly elevated levels of aluminum. These syndromes are sometimes seen in uremic patients, especially children, who have not been exposed to contaminated dialysate or intravenous fluids (Committee on Nutrition, 1986). In these cases, the source of aluminum appears to be aluminum–containing phosphate binder that are used to treat the hyperphosphatemia in uremics (Committee on Nutrition).

Often individuals at risk of developing these syndromes will have elevated serum levels of aluminum (Alfrey, 1986). Methodological problems make definition of normal serum aluminum levels difficult but generally serum aluminum levels <10 µg/l are considered normal (Versieck and Cornelis, 1980; Adan et al., 1986). Desferroxamine infusion tests have also been used to diagnose aluminum intoxication in uremic patients (Alfrey, 1986). A large increase in plasma aluminum levels (>700 µg Al/l) after a single injection of desferroxamine is considered evidence of an excessive body load of aluminum.

Although some elderly experience renal failure, dialysis osteodystrophy and dialysis encephalopathy are not the primary reasons for scientific interest in aluminum metabolism among the elderly. The intense interest in aluminum metabolism among the elderly is related to the observation by several investigators that aluminum accumulated in the brains of patients with Alzheimer's disease (Crapper et al., 1973; Perl and Brody, 1980; Perl, 1985). Similarly, the brains of patients with amyotrophic lateral sclerosis with parkinsonism dementia in Guam (ALS–PD) were found to contain elevated levels of aluminum (Perl et al., 1982; Garruto et al., 1986).

The hypothesis that aluminum is part of the etiology of either of these degenerative neurological syndromes is controversial (Wisnewski et al., 1985; Katzman, 1986; Lewin, 1987). Several investigators have been unable to demonstrate that the brains of patients with Alzheimer's

disease contained elevated concentrations of aluminum
(McDermott et al., 1979; Markesbery et al., 1981; Wisnewski
et al., 1985) but these investigators, however, noted that
aluminum tended to accumulate in brains with age (McDermott
et al., 1979; Markesbery et al., 1981).

The pathology of dialysis dementia is different from that
observed in Alzheimer's disease. In dialysis dementia,
aluminum tends to accumulate in the cytoplasm of cells;
there is no specific histopathology; and aluminum
accumulates in other tissues besides the brain (Wisniewski
et al., 1985; Alfrey, 1986). In Alzheimer's disease,
aluminum tends to accumulate in the nucleus of cells (Perl
and Brody, 1980; Perl, 1985); there are characteristic
neurofibrillary tangles (Katzman, 1986); and serum aluminum
levels are not elevated (Shore et al., 1980).

Other evidence against aluminum being the sole cause of
Alzheimer's disease is provided by studies with animal
models. Animal, which have been injected with aluminum, do
not develop all the symptoms of Alzheimer's disease, i.e.
the dramatic reduction in brain choline acetyltransferase
activity (Hetnarski et al., 1980; Coyle et al., 1983).
Moreover, histologically the neurofibrillary tangles induced
in animals by aluminum differ somewhat from those observed
in brains of patients with Alzheimer's disease (Wisniewski
et al., 1985).

Gajdusek (1985) has hypothesized that the etiology of
Alzheimer's disease and other dementia could vary somewhat
among patients. Any factor (i.e. trauma, subviral pathogen
or aluminum) that interfered with the axonal transport of
10 nm neurofilaments down axons could lead to deformation of
the neurofilament and ultimately the formation of the
neurofibrillary tangles and the neuritic or amyloid plaques
that histologically characterize the syndromes. Moreover,
Yase (1972) and Gajdusek (1984) have hypothesized that
aluminum from dietary sources was the primary cause of
ALS-PD in Guam. Furthermore, they suggested that the
consumption of native diets that were low in calcium and
magnesium promoted absorption and retention of dietary
aluminum.

Aluminum Metabolism

Evaluation of these hypotheses and any real assessment of
the importance of aluminum toxicity to the elderly requires
knowledge of aluminum metabolism. Unfortunately, data are
limited. Balance techniques do not appear to be sensitive
enough to monitor aluminum retention and absorption in
traditional ways (Ganrot, 1986; Greger, 1987). No
radioactive or stable isotopes of aluminum are usable as
tracers. However, new insights into aluminum metabolism
have been gained during the last ten years.

Urine, not bile, is believed to be the major excretory
route for aluminum (Kovalchik et al., 1978). Moreover,
urinary excretion of aluminum and serum levels of aluminum
have been found to be responsive to changes in dietary
intake of aluminum by young men (Greger and Baier, 1983).
Thus Ganrot (1986) suggested that absorption of aluminum
could be estimated on the basis of urinary aluminum losses.

Unfortunately, Greger et al. (1988) found recently that
although serum levels of aluminum were elevated, urinary
excretion of aluminum by thirteen postmenopausal women was
not changed when they consumed 1000 mg supplemental aluminum
hydroxide daily for several weeks. This may reflect the
form of the aluminum and the total dietary milieu; it may
also reflect the age of subjects. Other investigators have
not attempted to compare urinary excretion of aluminum by
young and elderly adults.

Aluminum, in at least trace amounts, has been found in
most tissues of humans and animals (Sorensen et al., 1974).
Several investigators have noted that aluminum tends to
accumulate in a number of tissues with age but no one has
systematically evaluated the effect of age on serum aluminum
levels (McDermott et al., 1979; Markesbery et al., 1981;
Ganrot, 1986). However, we observed that postmenopausal
women tended to have higher serum aluminum levels than young
adult males (Greger et al., 1988).

The effects of age on serum aluminum levels and the body
aluminum load need to be evaluated further. The gut may not
be the most logical organ system to study. Although Katz
et al. (1987) have observed the guts of rats become more
permeable to large molecules with age, investigators have
generally observed that absorption of minerals declined or

remained constant among the elderly (Heaney et al., 1982). Thus effects of age on the gut are not apt to increase the sensitivity of humans to aluminum exposure.

In contrast, the decline in renal function observed with age would promote aluminum accumulation (Lindeman, 1984). Greger and Donnaubauer (1986) observed that aluminum turnover in tissues was very rapid in young growing rats. Bone aluminum levels returned to control levels within one week after aluminum was removed from the diet. In contrast, removal of aluminum from the tissues of uremics is generally a slow process (Alfrey, 1986; Nebeker and Coburn, 1986). No one has studied aluminum retention in older animals or animals in which tissue turnover was decreased by disease states other than renal failure. This should be a focus in future studies on aluminum metabolism in the elderly.

SUMMARY

Research on the metabolism of trace elements by elderly individuals is limited. There are many exciting possibilities and hypotheses. But much work needs to be done to assess nutritional status in regard to trace elements of elderly individuals and to define "optimal" nutritional status.

ACKNOWLEDGMENT

The author appreciates the support of the College of Agricultural and Life Sciences, University of Wisconsin, Madison, WI, project No. 2623.

REFERENCES

Abdulla M, Jägerstad M, Norden A, Quist I, Svensson S (1977). Dietary intake of electrolytes and trace elements in the elderly. Nutr Metab 21 (Suppl 1), 41–44.
Adan L, Huinline BW, Jackison DA (1986). The importance of accurate and precise aluminum levels. New Engl J Med 313:1609.
Alfrey AC (1986) Aluminum. In Mertz W (ed): "Trace Elements in Human and Animal Nutrition," 5th Edition, Orlando FL: Academic Press, pp 399–414.

Anderson BM, Gibson RS, Sabry JH (1981). The iron and zinc status of long-term vegetarian women. Am J Clin Nutr 34:1042-1048.

Askari A, Long CL, Blakemore WS (1979). Urinary zinc, copper, nitrogen, and potassium losses in response to trauma. J Parenteral and Enteral Nutr 3:151-156.

Askari A, Long CL, Blakemore WS (1980). Zinc, copper and parenteral nutrition in cancer. A review. J Parenteral and Enteral Nutr 4:561-571.

Bales CW, Steinman LC, Freeland-Graves JH, Stone JM, Young RK (1986). The effect of age on plasma zinc uptake and taste acuity. Am J Clin Nutr 44:664-669.

Betts NM, Vivian VM. (1984). The dietary intake of noninstitutionalized elderly. J Nutr Elderly. 3(4):3-11.

Bogden JD Oleske JM, Munves EM, Lavenhar MA, Bruening K, Kemp FW, Holding KJ, Denny TN, Louria DB (1987). Zinc and immunocompetence in the elderly; baseline data on zinc nutriture and immunity in unsupplemented subjects. Am J Clin Nutr 46:101-109.

Brooks CB, Cummings LP (1984). Zinc and copper levels in hair, fingernails and plasma of elderly persons based on selected health conditions. J Nutr Elderly 3(4):27-38.

Bunker VW, Lawson MS, Delves HT, Clayton BE (1982). Metabolic balance studies for zinc and nitrogen in healthy elderly subjects. Human Nutr: Clinical Nutr 36:213-221.

Bunker VW, Hinks LJ, Lawson MS, Clayton BE (1984). Assessment of zinc and copper status of healthy elderly people using metabolic balance studies and measurement of leukocyte concentrations. Am J Clin Nutr 40:1096-1102.

Bunker VW, Hinks LJ, Stansfield MF, Lawson MS, Clayton BE (1987). Metabolic balance studies for zinc and copper in housebound elderly people and the relationship between zinc balance and leukocyte zinc concentrations. Am J Clin Nutr 46:353-359.

Burke, DM, De Micco FJ, Taper LJ, Ritchey SJ (1981). Copper and zinc utilization in elderly adults. J Gerontol 36:558-563.

Chandra RK (1984). Excessive intake of zinc impairs immune responses. J Am Med Assoc 252:1443-1446.

Chooi MK, Todd JK, Boyd ND (1976). Influence of age and sex on plasma zinc levels in normal and diabetic individuals. Nutr Metab 20:135-142.

Cohen IK, Schechter PJ, Henkin RI (1973). Hypogeusia, anorexia, and altered zinc metabolism following thermal burn. J Am Med Assoc 223:914-916.

Cohen DI, Illowsky B, Linder MC (1979). Altered copper

absorption in tumor–bearing and estrogen–treated rats. Am J Physiol 2363:E309–E315.

Committee on Nutrition. (1986). Aluminum toxicity in infants and children. Pediatrics 78:1150–1154.

Cooper RM, Bilask MA, Zubek JP (1959). The effect of age on taste sensitivity. J Gerontol 14:56–58.

Coyle JT, Price DL, DeLong MR (1983). Alzheimer's disease. A disorder of cortical cholinergic innervation. Science 219:1184–1190.

Crapper DR, Krishnan SS, Dalton AJ (1973). Brain aluminum distribution in Alzheimer's disease and experimental neurofibrillary degeneration. Science 180:511–513.

Croswell SC, Lei KY (1985). Effect of copper deficiency on the apolipoprotein E–rich high density lipoproteins in rats. J Nutr 115:473–482.

Deering TB, Dickson ER, Fleming CR, Geall MG, McCall JT, Baggenstoss AH (1977). Effect of D–penicillamine on copper retention in patients with primary biliary cirrhosis. Gastroenterology 71:1208–1212.

Denko CW, Gabriel P (1981). Age and sex related levels of albumin, ceruloplasmin, α, antitrypsin, α, acid glycoprotein, and transferrin. Ann Clin Lab Sci 11:63–68.

Duchateau J, Delepesse G, Vrijens R, Collet H (1981). Beneficial effect of oral zinc supplementation on the immune response of old people. Am J Med 70:1001–1004.

Fell GS, Fleck A, Cuthbertson DP, Queen K, Morrison C, Bessent RG, Hussain SL (1973). Urinary zinc levels as an indication of muscle catabolism. Lancet I:280–282.

Finley EB, Cerklewski FL (1983). Influence of ascorbic acid supplementation on copper status in young adult men. Am J Clin Nutr 37:553–556.

Fisher S, Hendricks DG, Mahoney AW (1978). Nutritional assessment of senior rural Utahns by biochemical and physical measurements. Am J Clin Nutr 31:667–672.

Flint DM, Wahlquist ML, Smith TJ, Parish AE (1981). Zinc and protein status in the elderly. J Human Nutr 35:287–295.

Food and Nutrition Board. (1980). "Recommended Dietary Allowances" 9th edition. Washington DC: National Academy of Sciences.

Fordyce EJ, Forbes RM, Robbins KR, Erdman JW Jr. (1987). Phytate X calcium/zinc molar ratios: Are they predictive of zinc bioavailability. J Food Sci 52:440–444.

Fosmire GJ, Manuel PA, Smiciklas-Wright H (1984). Dietary intake and zinc status of an elderly rural population. J Nutr Elderly 4(1):19–30.

Fraker PJ, Gershwin ME, Good RA, Prasad A (1986).
  Interrelationships between zinc and immune function.
  Federation Proceed. 45:1474-1479.
Fulwood R, Johnson CL, Bryner JD, Gunter EW, McGrath CR
  (1982). "Hematological and Nutritional Biochemistry
  Reference Data for Persons 6 Months - 74 Years of Age:
  United States, 1976-80." DHHS Publ No (PHS) 83-1682,
  Washington DC.: Dept. of Health and Human Services.
Gajdusek DC (1984). Calcium deficiency induced secondary
  hyperparathyroidism and resultant CNS deposition of
  calcium and other metallic cations as the cause of ALS and
  PD in high incidence among Auyu and Jakai people in West
  New Guinea. In Chen KM, Yase Y (eds): "Amyotrophic
  Lateral Sclerosis in Asia and Oceania," National Taiwan
  Univ, pp 145-155.
Gajdusek DC (1985). Hypothesis: Interference with axonal
  transport of neurofilament as a common pathogenetic
  mechanism in certain diseases of the central nervous
  system. New Engl J Med 312:714-719.
Ganrot PO (1986). Metabolism and possible health effects
  of aluminum. Environ Health Persp 65:363-441.
Garofalo JA, Ashikari H, Lesser ML, Menendez-Botet C,
  Cunningham-Rundles S, Schwartz MK, Good RA (1980). Serum
  zinc, copper and the Cu/Zn ratio in patients with benign
  and malignant breast lesions. Cancer 46:2682-2685.
Garruto RM, Swyt C, Yanagihara R, Fiori CE, Gajdusek DC
  (1986). Intraneuronal co-localization of silicon with
  calcium and aluminum in amyotrophic lateral sclerosis and
  parkinsonism with dementia of Guam. New Engl J Med
  315:711-712.
Gibson RA, Anderson BM, Sabry JH (1983). The trace metal
  status of a group of post-menopausal vegetarians. J Am
  Dietet Assoc 82:246-250.
Greger JL (1977). Dietary intake and nutritional status in
  regard to zinc of institiutionalized aged. J Gerontol
  32:549-553.
Greger JL (1982). Effects of phosphorus-containing
  compounds on iron and zinc utilization: A review of the
  literature. In Kies C (ed): "Nutritional Bioavailability
  of Iron," Washington, DC: American Chemical Society, pp
  107-120.
Greger JL (1985). Aluminum content of the American diet.
  Food Technol 39:73,73,76,78-80.
Greger JL (1986). Trace minerals. In Chen NH (ed):
  "Nutritional Aspects of Aging," Vol. 1, Boca Raton, FL:
  CRC Press, pp 255-278.

Greger JL (1987). Aluminum and tin. Wld Rev Nutr Diet 54:255–285.

Greger JL, Baier MJ (1983). Excretion and retention of low or moderate levels of aluminum by human subjects. Fd Chem Toxicol 21:473–477.

Greger JL, Donnaubauer SE (1986). Retention of aluminum in the tissues of rats after the discontinuation of oral exposure to aluminum. Fd Chem Toxicol 24:1331–1334.

Greger, JL, Geissler AH (1978). Effect of zinc supplementation on taste acuity of the aged. Am J Clin Nutr 31:633–637.

Greger JL, Krashoc CL, Nielsen FH, Mullen LM (1988). Aluminum metabolism in post–menopausal women. J Trace Elements Expt Med (In press).

Greger JL, Sciscoe BA (1977). Zinc nutriture of elderly participants in an urban feeding program. J Am Dietet Assoc 70:37–41.

Greger JL, Snedeker SM (1980). Effect of dietary protein and phosphorus levels on the utilization of zinc, copper and manganese by adult males. J Nutr 110:2243–2253.

Greger JL, Zaikis SC, Abernathy RP, Bennett OA, Huffman J (1978). Zinc, nitrogen, copper, iron and manganese balance in adolescent females fed two levels of zinc. J Nutr 108:1449–1456.

Gregoriadis GC, Apostolidis NS, Romanos AN, Paradellis TP (1982). Postoperative changes in serum copper value. Surg Gynecol Obstet 154:217–221.

Haeger K, Lanner E, Magnusson PO (1974). Oral zinc sulfate in the treatment of venous leg ulcers. In Pories WJ, Strain WH, Hsu JM, Woosley RL (eds): "Clinical applications of zinc metabolism," Springfield: Charles C. Thomas Publisher, pp 158–167.

Hallböök T, Lanner E. (1972). Serum–zinc and healing of venous leg ulcers. Lancet II:780.

Hambidge KM, Casey CE, Krebs NF Zinc. (1986). In Mertz W (ed): "Trace elements in human and animal nutrition," 5th ed. Orlando, FL: Academic Press pp 1–137.

Harvey PW, Allen KGD (1981). Decreased plasma lecithin: Cholesterol acyltransferase activity in copper–deficient rats. J Nutr 111:1855–1858.

Heaney RP, Gallagher JC, Johnston CC, Neer R, Parfitt AM, Whedon GD (1982). Calcium nutrition and bone health in the elderly. Am J Clin Nutr 36:986–1013.

Henkin RI, Patten BM, Re PK, Bonzert DA (1975). A syndrome of acute zinc loss. Arch Neurol 32:745–751.

Hetnarski B, Wisniewski HM, Iqbal K, Dziedzic J, Lajtha A

(1980). Central cholinergic activity in aluminum-induced neurofibrillary degeneration. Ann Neurol 7:489-490.

Husain SL, Bessent RG. Oral zinc sulfate in the treatment of leg ulcers. (1974) In Pories WJ, Strain WH, Hsu JM, Woosley RL (eds): "Clinical Applications of zinc metabolism," Springfield: Charles C. Thomas Publisher, pp 168-178.

Hutton CW, Hayes-Davis RB (1983). Assessment of the zinc nutritional status of selected elderly subjects. J Am Dietet Assoc 82:148-153.

Johnson MA, Baier MJ, Greger JL (1982). Effects of dietary tin on zinc, copper, iron, manganese and magnesium metabolism of adult males. Am J Clin Nutr 35:1332-1338.

Karp BF, Roboz M, Linder MC (1986). Regulation of ceruloplasmin and copper turnover by estrogens and tumors in the rat. J Nutr Growth Cancer 3:47-55.

Katz D, Hollander D, Said HM, Dadufalza V (1987). Aging-associated increase in intestinal permeability to polyethylene glycol 900. Dig Dis & Sci 32:285-288.

Katzman R. (1986). Alzheimer's disease. New Engl J Med 314:964-973.

King SW, Savory J, Wells MR (1981). The clinical biochemistry of aluminum. CRC Crit Rev Clin Lab Sci 14:1-20.

Klevay LM (1984). The role of copper, zinc and other chemical elements in ischemic heart disease. In Rennert OW, Chan WY (eds): "Metabolism of Trace Metals in Man," Vol. I Boca Raton, FL: CRC Press, pp 129-152.

Klevay LM, Bistrian BR, Fleming R, Neumann CG (1987). Hair analysis in clinical and experimental medicine. Am J Clin Nutr 46:233-236.

Klevay LM, Reck SJ, Barcome DF (1979). Evidence of dietary copper and zinc deficiencies. J Am Med Assoc 241:1916-1918.

Klevay LM, Reck SJ, Jacob RA, Logan GM Jr, Munoz JM, Sandstead HH (1980). The human requirement for copper, 1. Healthy men fed conventional, American diets. Am J Clin Nutr 33:45-50.

Kovalchik MT, Kaehney WD, Hegg AP, Jackson AT, Alfrey AC (1978). Aluminum kinetics during hemodialysis. J Lab Clin Med 92:712-720.

Krebs JM, Schneider VS, LeBlanc AD (1988). Zinc, copper and nitrogen balances during bed rest and fluoride supplementation in healthy adult males. Am J Clin Nutr 47:509-514.

Law BWC, Klevay LM (1981). Plasma lecithin: Cholesterol

acyltransferase in copper–deficient rats. J Nutr 111:1698–1703.

Lefevre M, Keen CL, Lönnerdal B, Hurley LS, Schneeman BO (1986). Copper deficiency–induced hypercholesterolemia: Effects on HDL subfractions and hepatic lipoprotein receptor activity in the rat. J Nutr 116:1735–1746.

Lei KY (1978). Oxidation, excretion and tissue distribution of [26^{14}C]cholesterol in copper–deficient rats. J Nutr 108:232–237.

Lei KY (1983). Alterations in plasma lipid, lipoprotein and apolipoprotein concentrations in copper–deficient rats. J Nutr 113:2178–2183.

Lewin R (1987). Environmental hypothesis for brain diseases strengthened by new data. Science 237:483–484.

Life Sciences Research Office (1984). "Assessment of the zinc nutritional status of the U.S. population based on data collected in the second National Health and Nutrition Examination Survey, 1976–1980." Bethesda, MD: Federation of American Societies for Experimental Biology, 62pp.

Lifschitz MD, Henkin RI (1971). Circadian variation in copper and zinc in man. J Appl Physiol 31:88–92.

Lindeman RD, Clark ML, Colmore JP (1971). Influence of age and sex on plasma and red–cell zinc concentrations. J Gerontol 26:358–363.

Lindeman RD (1984). Changes in kidney function with age. Geriatric Med Today 3(5):41–43,45,47.

Lione A (1985). Aluminum intake from non–prescription drugs and sucralfate. Gen Pharmacol 16:223–228.

Markesbery WR, Ehmann WD, Hossain TIM, Alauddin M, Goodin DR (1981). Instrumental neutron activation analysis of brain aluminum in Alzheimer's disease and aging. Ann Neurol 10:511–516.

McDermott JR, Smith I, Iqbal K, Wisniewski HM (1979) Brain aluminum in aging and Alzheimer disease. Neurology 29:809–814.

McGandy RB, Russell RM, Hartz SC, Jacob RA, Tannenbaum S, Peters H, Sahyoun N, Otradovec CL (1986). Nutritional status survey of noninstitutionalized elderly; energy and nutrient intakes from three–day dietary records and nutrient supplements. Nutr Res 6:785–798.

Mills BJ, Broghamer WL, Higgins PJ, Lindeman RD (1984). Inhibition of tumor growth by zinc depletion of rats. J Nutr 114:746–752.

Milne DB, Omaye ST, Amos WH Jr. (1981). Effect of ascorbic acid on copper and cholesterol in adult cynomolgus monkeys fed a diet marginal in copper. Am J Clin Nutr

34:2389-2393.

Minkel DT, Dolhum PJ, Calhoun BL, Saryan LA, Petering DH (1979). Zinc deficiency and growth of Ehrlich ascites tumor. Cancer Res 39:2451-2456.

Morley JB (1986). Nutritional status of the elderly. Am J Med 81:679-695.

Murphy P, Wadiwala I, Sharland DE, Rai GS (1985). Copper and zinc levels in "healthy: and "sick" elderly. J Am Geriatrics Soc 33:847-849.

Nebeker HG, Coburn JW (1986). Aluminum and renal osteodystrophy. Ann Review Med 37:79-95.

Paterson PG, Lee E, Christensen DA, Robertson D (1985). Zinc levels or hospitalized elderly. J Am Dietet Assoc 85:186-191.

Pennington JT, Calloway DH (1973). Copper content of foods. J Am Dietet Assoc 63:143-153.

Pennington JAT, Young BE, Wilson DB, Johnson RD, Vanderveen JE (1986). Mineral content of foods and total diets: The selected minerals in foods survey, 1982 to 1984. J Am Dietet Assoc 86:876-897.

Perl DP (1985). Relationship of aluminum to Alzheimer's disease. Environ Health Persp 63:149-153.

Perl DP, Brody AR (1980). Alzheimer's disease: X-ray spectrometric evidence of aluminum accumulation in neurofibrillary tangle-bearing neurons. Science 208:297-299.

Perl DP, Gajdusek DC, Garruto R, Yanagihara RT, Gibbs CJ Jr. (1982). Intraneuronal aluminum accumulation in amyotrophic lateral sclerosis and parkinsonism-dementia of Guam. Science 217:1053-1055.

Petering HG, Murthy L, O'Flaherty E (1977). Influence of dietary copper and zinc on rat lipid metabolism. J Agric Food Chem 25:1105-1109.

Prasad A (1986). Spectrum of human zinc deficiency. First Meeting of the International Society for Trace Element Research in Humans, Dec. 8-12, 1986. Palm Springs, CA, Abstract 1.

Prasad AS (1979). "Zinc in Human Nutrition." Boca Raton, FL: CRC Press, pp 17-30.

Rao KMK (1982). Age-related differential effects of zinc on concanavalin A-induced capping of human lymphocytes. Exptl Gerontol 17:205-211.

Reding P, Duchateau J, Bataille C (1984). Oral zinc supplementation improves hepatic encephalopathy. Lancet I:493-494.

Reiser S, Smith JC, Mertz W, Holbrook JT, Scholfield DJ,

Powell AS, Canfield WK, Canary JJ (1985). Indices of copper status in humans consuming a typical American diet containing either fructose or sucrose. Am J Clin Nutr 42:242-251.

Roe DA (1976). "Drug-Induced Nutritional Deficiences." Westport: AVI Publishing Co, pp 145-153.

Sahyoun NR, Otradovec CL, Hartz SC, Jacob RA, Peters H, Russell RM, McGandy RB (1988). Dietary intakes and biochemical indicators of nutritional status in an elderly, institutionalized population. Am J Clin Nutr 47:524-533.

Sandstead HH (1982a). Availability of zinc and its requirements in human subjects. In Prasad AS (ed): "Clinical, Biochemical, and Nutritional Aspects of Trace Elements," New York: Alan R. Liss, pp 83-101.

Sandstead HH (1982b). Copper bioavailability and requirements. Am J Clin Nutr 35:809-814.

Sandstead HH, Henriksen LK, Greger JL, Prasad AS, Good RS (1982). Zinc nutriture in the elderly in relation to taste acuity, immune response and wound healing. Am J Clin Nutr 36:1046-1059.

Sandstead HH, Munoz JM, Jacob RA, Klevay LM, Reck S, Logan GM Jr, Dintzis FR, Inglett GE, Shuey WC (1978). Influence of dietary fiber on trace element balance. Am J Clin Nutr 31:S180-S184.

Sandström B, Andersson H, Bosaeus I, Flakheden T, Goransson H, Melkersson M (1983). The effect of wheat bran on the intake of energy and nutrients and on serum mineral levels in constipated geriatric patients. Human Nutr: Clin Nutr 37C:295-300.

Schreurs WHP, Klosse JA, Muys T, Haesen JP (1982). Serum copper levels in relation to sex and age. Internat J Vit Nutr Res 52:68-74.

Science and Education Administration (1980). "Food and Nutrient Intakes of Individuals in 1 Day in the United States, Spring 1977." Prelim. Rep. No. 2. Washington DC: USDA.

Seligson FH (1980). Sodium intake, preference and taste acuity in elderly subjects before and after zinc supplementation. Unpublished manuscript.

Sempos CT, Greger JL, Johnson NE, Smith EL, Seyedabadi FM (1983). Levels of serum copper and magnesium in normotensives and untreated and treated hypertensives. Nutr Rep Intl 27:1013-1020.

Sempos CT, Johnson NE, Elmer PJ, Allington JK, Mathews ME (1982). A dietary survey of 14 Wisconsin nursing homes.

J Am Dietet Assoc 81:35-40.

Shore D, Millson M, Holtz JL, King SW, Bridge TP, Wyatt RJ (1980). Serum aluminum in primary degenerative dementia. Biol Psychiatry 15:971-977.

Solomons NW (1982). Biological availability of zinc in humans. Am J Clin Nutr 35:1048-1075.

Sorensen JRJ, Campbell IR, Tepper LB, Lingg RD (1974). Aluminum in the environment and human health. Environ Health Perspect 8:3-95.

Spencer H, Kramer L, Osis D (1982). Zinc balance in humans. In Prasad AS, (ed): "Clinical, Biochemical, and Nutritional Aspects of Trace Elements," New York: Alan R. Liss, pp 103-115.

Stiedemann M, Harrill I (1980). Relation of immunocompetence to selected nutrients in elderly women. Nutr Rep Intl 21:931-942.

Sullivan JF, Blotchy AJ, Jetton MM, Hahn HD Jr., Burch RE (1979). Serum levels of selenium calcium, copper, magnesium, manganese and zinc in various human diseases. J Nutr 109:1432-1437.

Thomas AJ, Bunker VW, Brennan E, Clayton BE (1986). The trace element content of hospital meals and potential low intake by elderly patients. Human Nutr: Appl Nutr 40A:440-446.

Turnlund J, Costa F, Margen S (1981). Zinc, copper, and iron balance in elderly men. Am J Clin Nutr 34:2641-2647.

Turnlund JR, Durkin N, Costa F, Margen S (1986). Stable isotope studies of zinc absorption and retention in young and elderly men. J Nutr 116:1239-1247.

Turnlund JR, Durkin N, Margen S (1984). Copper and iron absorption in young and elderly men. Am J Clin Nutr 39:664 (abstract).

Turnlund JR, Michel MC, Keyes WR, Schultz Y, Margen S (1982). Copper absorption in elderly men determined by using stable ^{65}Cu. Am J Clin Nutr 36:587-591.

Uaoy R, Castillo-Duran C, Fisberg M, Fernandez N, Valenzuela A (1985). Red cell superoxide dismutase activity as an index of human copper nutrition. J Nutr 115:1650-1655.

Underwood EJ (1977). "Trace Elements in Human and Animal Nutrition." Fourth edition. New York: Academic Press, pp 56-108, 430-433.

Ventura MT, Crollo R, Lasaracina E (1986). In vitro zinc correction of natural killer activity in the elderly. Clin Exp Immunol 64:223-224.

Versieck J, Cornelis R (1980). Measuring aluminum levels. New Engl J Med 302:468.

Vir SC, Love AHG (1979). Zinc and copper status of the elderly. Am J Clin Nutr 32:1472-1476.

Wagner PA, Bailey LB, Krista ML, Jernigan JA, Robinson JD, Cerda JJ (1981). Comparison of zinc and folacin status in elderly women from differing socioeconomic backgrounds. Nutr Res 1:565-569.

Wagner PA, Jernigan JA, Bailey LB, Nickens C, Brazzi GA (1983). Zinc nutriture and cell mediated immunity in the aged. Intl J Vit Nutr Res 53:94-101.

Wagner P, Krista ML, Bailey LB, Christakis GJ, Jernigan JA, Araujo PE, Appledorf H, Davis GC, Dinning JS (1980). Zinc status of elderly black Americans from urban low-income households. Am J Clin Nutr 33:1771-1777.

Weismann K, Wanscher B, Krakaver R (1978). Oral zinc therapy in geriatric patients with selected skin manifestations and a low plasma zinc level. Acta Dermat 58:157-161.

Welsh, SO, Marston RM (1982). Zinc levels of the US food supply - 1909-1980. Food Technol 36:70-76.

Wester PO. (1980). Tissue zinc at autopsy-relation to medication with diuretics. Acta Med Scand 208:269-271.

Wisniewski HM, Sturman JA, Shek JW, Iqbal K (1985). Aluminum and the central nervous system. J Environ Pathol Toxicol Oncol 6:1-8.

Yase Y (1972). The pathogenesis of amyotrophic lateral sclerosis. Lancet II:292-296.

Youssef AAR, Wood B, Baron DN (1983). Serum copper: A marker of disease activity in rheumatoid arthritis. J Clin Pathol 36:14-17.

Mineral Homeostasis in the Elderly, pages 201–204
© 1989 Alan R. Liss, Inc.

Research Summary:

SOME BIOCHEMICAL CONSEQUENCES OF ZINC DEFICIENCY IN MAN

P. Isaac Rabbani and Ananda S. Prasad

Wayne State University Department of Medicine,
Detroit and VA Medical Center, Allen Park,
Michigan, 48101

INTRODUCTION

The first human zinc deficiency (Zn def) syndrome was
recognized by Prasad et al. in 1961 and reported later (Prasad et al., 1963). Subsequently, Zn metabolism has been extensively investigated in both man and animals. These studies showed that Zn def can result from insufficient dietary
intake (Greger, 1977), certain disease states (Dodge and
Yassa, 1978), excessive excretion (Smith, 1977), prolonged
and unsupplemented parenteral nutrition (Kay and Tasman-
Jones, 1975), as well as intestinal malabsorption (Sandstead,
1973). Thus, in 1974 the Food and Nutrition Board of the
National Academy of Sciences first published a Recommended
Dietary Allowance (RDA) for Zn. However, a recent report
(Pennington et al., 1988) indicated that in some age-sex
groups, including older people, dietary Zn intake is below
the RDA level.

In a previous report (Rabbani et al., 1987) we described
a flexible dietary model for production of experimental Zn
def in man. The study indicated that the RDA for Zn may be
inadequate for vegetarians and older people. In the present
communication we describe some biochemical consequences of
the induced Zn def in the latest subject studied (a 58-year-
old man).

A 7-day semi-purified diet based on soy protein was fed
to the volunteer for 28 weeks (depletion phase: DP, 4.8 mg
Zn per day) followed by 20 weeks (wk) of the diet supplemented with 30 mg Zn per day (repletion phase: RP). Overall,

the subject received 2.7 mg Zn per day due to the elimination of 2 days of the planned high Zn menu and uneaten foods.
Blood was collected twice a month. Pancreatic juice was
collected at least twice during each phase. Details of the
experimental design and some analytical methods have been
described elsewhere (Rabbani et al., 1987).

RESULTS

After 20 wk of Zn depletion, the volunteer lost 200 mg
body Zn. This was accompanied by a significant decline in
plasma and lymphocyte Zn concentrations (Rabbani et al.,
1987). Plasma alkaline phosphatase, erythrocyte (RBC) and
lymphocyte nucleoside phosphorylase (Fig. 1), and RBC delta-
aminolevulonate dehydratase activities were decreased and
plasma ammonia increased significantly during Zn DP (Fig. 2).
However, all these parameters returned to normal upon 20 wk
of repletion with 30 mg Zn per day. While serum testosterone, neutrophil alkaline phosphatase activity and plasma BUN
(Fig. 2) were not affected by Zn depletion, they significantly increased after the Zn RP.

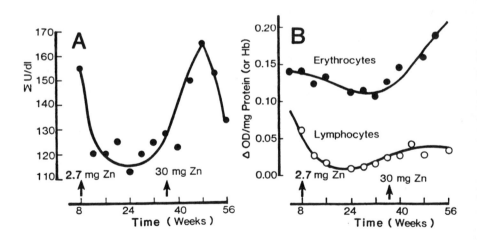

Figure 1. Effects of zinc depletion and repletion on activities of plasma alkaline phosphatase (A) and erythrocytes and
lymphocytes nucleoside phosphorylase (B) in a 59-year-old man.

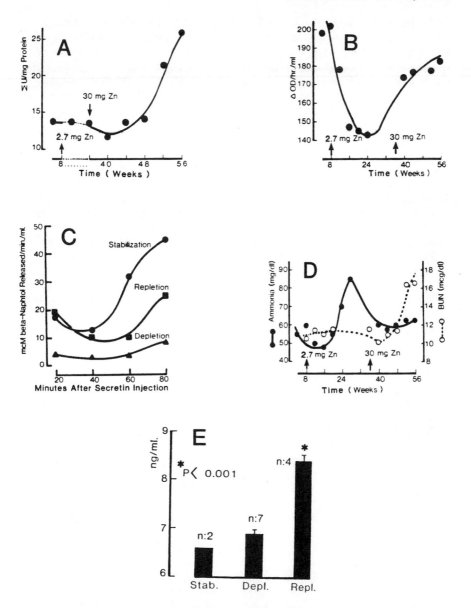

Figure 2. Effects of zinc depletion and repletion on activities of neutrophil alkaline phosphatase (A), RBC delta-aminolevulonate dehydratase (B), pancreatic carboxypeptidase-A (C), and concentrations of plasma ammonia and BUN (D), and serum testosterone (E) in a 58-year-old man.

We conclude that: (a) While mild, long-term Zn deficiency symptoms can be induced by dietary means without per-
manent effects, older subjects require more Zn for a longer
time to reverse these symptoms: (b) Older people may be at
higher risk of developing severe Zn deficiency and consequently becoming more vulnerable to disease of old age.

REFERENCES

Dodge JA, Yassa JG (1978). Zinc deficiency in a British
youth with cystic fibrosis. Br Med J 1:411.
Food and Nutrition Board: "Recommended dietary allowances.",
8th Ed, 1974. Washington, DC, National Academy of Sciences, National Research Council, pp 99-101.
Greger JL (1977). Dietary intake and nutritional status in
regard to zinc of institutionalized aged. J Geront 32:
549-553.
Kay RG, Tasman-Jones C (1975). Acute zinc deficiency in man
during intravenous alimentation. Aust NZ J Surg 45:325-
330.
Pennington JAT, Young BE, Wilson DB (1988). Nutritional
elements in U. S. diets: results from the Total Diet Study, 1982-1986. FDA, Center for Food Safety and Applied
Nutrition, Internal Report No. 88-120, Washington, DC.
USA.
Prasad AS, Halsted JA, Nadimi M (1961). Syndrome of iron
deficiency anemia, hepatosplemonegaly, hypogonadism,
dwarfism and geophagia. Am J Med 31:532-546.
Prasad AS, Schulert AR, Miale A, Jr, Farid Z, Sandstead HH
(1963). Zinc metabolism in patients with the syndrome of
iron deficiency anemia, hepatosplenomegaly, dwarfism and
hypogonadism. J Lab Clin Med 61:537-549.
Rabbani PI, Prasad AS, Tsai R, Harland BF, Fox MRS (1987).
Dietary model for production of experimental zinc deficien-
cy in man. Am J Clin Nutr 45:1514-1525.
Sandstead HH (1973). Zinc nutrition in the United States.
Am J Clin Nutr 26:1251-1260.
Smith JC, Jr (1977). Heritable hyperzincemia in humans. In
Brewer GJ, Prasad AS (eds): "Zinc Metabolism: Current
Aspects in Health and Disease", New York: Alan R. Liss,
pp 181-187.

COPING WITH THE EFFECTS OF CHRONIC ILLNESS AND AGE ON MINERAL STATUS

Mineral Homeostasis in the Elderly, pages 207–222
© *1989 Alan R. Liss, Inc.*

NUTRITIONAL REGULATION OF HOST DEFENSE
SYSTEMS: EMPHASIS ON TRACE MINERALS

Robert J. Cousins

Center for Nutritional Sciences

University of Florida, Gainesville, Florida

INTRODUCTION

Aging is as natural phenomenon as is the need to
acquire nutrients. Therefore, it is a natural extension
of inquiry to ponder the usefulness of dietary intake as
a medium to control or reverse this process. A corollary
axiom is that certain nutrients are particularly
beneficial in defending against disease. It is
understandable that with advancing age considerable
attention is placed on the role nutrients serve in
limiting the aging process and supporting host defense
mechanisms to combat disease.

At the present time some definite conclusions can be
drawn relative to the elderly, trace elements and host
defense based on epidemiological evidence. Only
recently, however, have isolated biochemical and
molecular data begun to provide a focus for a mechanistic
understanding of the complex phenomena involved. In this
short review, contemporary literature dealing with the
trace elements: copper, iron, selenium, and zinc will be
discussed from both mechanistic and observational levels
in an effort to increase discussion and interest in these
functions related to host defense.

TRACE ELEMENTS AND HOST DEFENSE

There is a substantial literature base to confirm
that trace elements have been the class of nutrients most

widely implicated in host defense processes. Relatively few studies have been devoted specifically related to the elderly. However, that may not be essential because it is with advancing age that degenerative disease places the greatest requisite burden on defense processes. Each of the four nutrients will be discussed individually from the epidemiological to the molecular level. An attempt will then be made to integrate information into the prospective of elderly subjects.

A common theme will be the role of cytokines in diseases associated with aging, i.e. atherosclerosis, arthritis and osteoporosis and how these mediators of systemic responses effect trace elements. Furthermore, each of the trace elements to be discussed, copper, iron, selenium and zinc, can be integrated into generalized antioxidant defense systems which are of particular concern in the elderly. In addition, both cell-mediated and hormonal immunity declines with age. Since these systems are particularly sensitive to trace element status antioxidant effects may again be implicated in the age-related decline in immunocompetence and perhaps age-related degenerative disease.

COPPER

The two metalloenzymes through which copper has a role in host defense are superoxide dismutase (EC 1.15.1.1) and ceruloplasmin (EC 1.14.3.1).

Superoxide dismutase, a 34 kDa protein is found in virtually all aerobic cells, but is particularly abundant in brain, heart, erythrocytes and liver (Halliwell, 1987). The cytosolic form contains 2 atoms each of copper and zinc. In cells, ferrous iron reacts with dioxygen to produce superoxide ion, $Fe(II) + O_2 \rightarrow Fe(III) + O_2^-$. Superoxide dismutase then catalyzes the conversion of O_2^- to H_2O_2 (Aust et al., 1985). Collectively these oxygen radicals produce the microbicidal oxidative activity of neutrophils, monocytes and macrophages (Halliwell, 1987). However, it is generally believed to comprise oxidative stress in cells and tissues. Nutritional restriction of copper has been shown repeatedly to decrease the activity of the enzyme (reviewed in Fields et al., 1984). This decrease probably relates to lack of copper incorporation into the apoenzyme during translation. It is generally believed that superoxide dismutase is an inducible system by agents such as endotoxin (Crapo and Tierney, 1974). Since genes for the enzyme are being cloned, new information on the relationship of this dismutase to host defense against oxidative stress will be forthcoming.

Considerably more is known about ceruloplasmin in terms of its nutritional significance albeit its place within host defense is not clear. The enzyme is large, 132 kDa with four copper atoms per molecule. Many functions for the protein have been described including plasma copper transport to tissue sites for uptake and as a serum antioxidant against superoxide ion (Frieden, 1986). The latter proposal has been criticized from the standpoint that superoxide dismutase displays greater activity toward superoxide ion. However, it has been suggested that the presence of ceruloplasmin in serum rather than erythrocytes may indicate an extracellular antioxidant function for this secreted enzyme (Cousins, 1985).

Recently the synthesis of ceruloplasmin has been closely investigated. Synthesis is stimulated by immunostimulatory agents such as interleukin-1 (Barber and Cousins, 1988). Induction is independent of copper, but copper is required for oxidase activity and presumably function. In dietary copper deficiency, ceruloplasmin activity is decreased and is diagnostic of the condition (reviewed in Cousins, 1985). Genes for human and rat ceruloplasmin have been cloned recently (Koschinsky et al., 1986; Aldred et al., 1987) and ELISA assays have been developed to measure the protein in plasma (DiSilvestro and David, 1986; DiSilvestro et al, 1988). This should stimulate interest in this area. For example, Aldred et al. (1987) have shown the presence of ceruloplasmin mRNA in cerebrospinal fluid. Since the protein acts as an oxidase for amines with neurotransmitter action, they suggest a function for ceruloplasmin in the central nervous system. The elderly are particularly susceptible to neurological problems, e.g. senility and Alzheimer's Disease. Therefore, adequate copper levels to insure optimum ceruloplasmin oxidase activity may be very important, particularly in the elderly.

The increase in plasma ceruloplasmin observed during infection, tissue injury and antigenic stimulation is signalled by interleukin-1 (Barber and Cousins, 1988). This cytokine in turn stimulates T cells to produce interleukin-6 (β_2-interferon) which probably is the actual mediator (Dinarello, 1987). Since T cell-mediated functions appear to decline with age (Blumberg and Meydani, 1986), it is possible that the induction of ceruloplasmin by cytokines may be concomitantly compromised. Ceruloplasmin is also necessary for ferroxidase active to convert Fe(II) to Fe(III). This decreases the pool of Fe(II) available to react with H_2O_2 and produce hydroxyl radicals (2). The latter reaction ($Fe(II) + H_2O_2 \rightarrow \cdot OH + Fe(III) + OH^-$) is responsible for lipid peroxidation and oxidative damage to DNA. During a reduction in copper intake, the potential for Fe(II)-related hepatic damage is greater since iron is not released from the liver. Furthermore, since bilirubin binds copper in the gastrointestinal tract (Stocker and Ames, 1987), it may be necessary for ceruloplasmin to closely control the return of copper to hepatocytes for excretion.

Dietary copper deficiency increases lipid peroxidation based on ethane evolution, a very sensitive method (Lawrence and Jenkinson, 1987). Ceruloplasmin activity was also decreased. In contrast, Kubow et al (1986) did not observe an effect of this deficiency on spontaneous, microsomal free radical production. The evidence is in favor of increased lipid peroxidation in copper deficiency, an occurrence that is also observed during aging.

Prohaska et al. (1983) have shown reduced splenic T cell function in copper deficient mice. This was correlated to reduced plasma ceruloplasmin (Prohaska & Lukasewycz (1981). Reduced microbicidal activity could be related to superoxide dismutase which is needed to produce H_2O_2. Chandra (1988) has reviewed the evidence for an immunological role for copper.

IRON

The beneficial and deleterious effects of iron have been repeatedly emphasized (Aust et al., 1985; Halliwell,

1987). The beneficial aspects are of course related to hematopoiesis. This does not appear to change with age, but the response of the hematopoietic system may change with age. The other beneficial aspect of iron is that it is needed for bactericidal activity in cell mediated host defense.

The iron status of elderly individuals is usually not low enough to produce deficiency. However, lower iron status is associated with impaired cell-mediated immunity, response to antigenic challenge, cytokine production and macrophage migration (reviewed in Heresi, 1986). These could involve decreased DNA synthesis, myeloperoxidase activity and hydroxyl radical formation among others. For example, lactoferrin helps maintain natural killer activity of monocytes. Similarly, transferrin may aid in iron uptake by T cells (Weinberg, 1986). This process is stimulated by IL-2 and induction of transferrin receptors on T cells. Overall suboptimal iron status may place the elderly at some risk to infection.

Iron is a two edged sword, with respect to host defense. While iron is required to generate superoxide radicals and to participate in iron-requiring, beneficial processes, it is a toxic trace element that must be carefully controlled. The storage of iron is tightly controlled by ferritin synthesis by iron-controlled translational regulation (Zahringer et al.,1976) through a cis-acting iron-responsive element in ferritin mRNA (Hentze et al.,1987). Circulating iron is controlled in part through iron-sensitive transcriptional regulation of transferrin (Idzerda et al.,1986). The latter is an increased acute phase response to certain host defense mediators.

Weinberg (1986) and others have placed considerable attention on the detrimental effects of excess iron. Pathogenic microorganisms avidly acquire iron through secreted iron chelators called siderophores. It is proposed that as the iron saturation of transferrin increases so does the ability of these invading organisms to acquire iron. He believes that lowering the iron content of the diet, induction of interleukin-1, elevation of body temperature or administration of a specific iron chelator of high binding capacity will

prevent the incidence of infection. A rationale he uses
is that early in the infectious process the plasma iron
concentration is reduced (Dinarello., 1987). This could
represent an iron withdrawal system. Alternatively, the
hypoferremic response could be a manifestation of iron
uptake by granulocyte lactoferrin (Goldblum et al, 1987).

The influence of excess iron on tissue damage and
neoplasia also is relevant to host defense and the
elderly. Weinberg (1986) has proposed that excess iron
contributes to carcinogenesis. This could occur in many
ways: 1) a generalized increase in iron-generated
hydroxyl radicals could increase tissue damage including
the genome; 2) Cerutti (1985) has theorized about
prooxidant genes and how they relate to tumor promotion.
Iron-related lipid peroxidation could contribute at this
level; 3) iron is required for the P-450 system and
radicals generated in this way could contribute to
cellular damage including the DNA.

Generalized lipid peroxidation associated with aging
and oxidative stress have been discussed repeatedly over
the years as has the value of antioxidants. Indeed,
convincing arguments can be made to relate tissue
peroxidation to longevity and aging (Cutler, 1985;
Blumberg and Meydani, 1986). In this regard, consumption
of excess iron as supplements remains controversial
because this practice will increase iron levels of the
gastrointestinal tract and maximize systemic iron status.
Nevertheless, supplemental iron is consumed by large
numbers of individuals including the elderly in developed
countries.

SELENIUM

There is a large volume of literature relating
selenium to both lipid peroxidation and neoplasia. A
negative correlation exists between selenium status and
cancer incidence (Ip, 1985; Milner, 1985; Burk, 1986).

A major breakthrough in our understanding of these
relationships came with the discovery that one form of
glutathione peroxidase (EC 1.11.1.9) is
selenium-dependent (Rotruck et al., 1973). It was rapidly
developed into a cogent mechanism where lipid peroxides

produced by free radicals are enzymatically converted to hydroxy acids by glutathione peroxidase (Chow and Tappel, 1974). Activity of this 90 kDa metalloenzyme is sensitive to dietary selenium status in many tissues including neutrophils and macrophages (Serfass and Ganther, 1975, 1976). Activity appears to be sensitive to copper status as well (Fields et al., 1984), but the mechanism for the effect is unknown. The effect of aging on glutathione peroxidase is not clear. It is higher in older rats but lower in elderly human populations compared to appropriate counterparts in each case (reviewed in Blumberg and Meydani, 1986).

Antitumor properties of selenium have been described (LeBoeuf and Hoekstra, 1985). Data has been presented to show that selenium changes cellular GSSG/GSH ratios. This has the effect of increasing the G_1 phase of cells. The elevated GSSG may decrease protein synthesis in cells by inhibiting initiation factor 2. However, selenium is required for induction of cytochrome P-450 (Newman and Guzelian, 1982). This latter observation suggests that under some conditions selenium could act as a tumor promoter. Levander (1987) has reviewed the evidence for the protective effects of dietary selenium.

ZINC

The contribution of zinc to host defense mechanisms has received considerable attention during the past decade. Two main systems seem to be operative. One involves apponent multiple functions in the immune system. The other involves antioxidant properties attributed to zinc ions, zinc complexes or zinc metallothionein. A hypothesis on aging as an intracellular zinc deficiency has been proposed (Garfinkel, 1986).

Extensive reviews on the relationship of zinc to immune function are available (Fraker et al., 1986; Chandra, 1988). Congenital zinc malabsorption in cattle (Adema Disease) and humans (acrodermatitis Enteropathica) lead to abnormal immune responses. Both are correctable with supplemental zinc. In contrast to these hereditary syndromes, zinc deficiency may be a primary or secondary factor in decreased immunity associated with protein-energy malnutrition.

A major breakthrough in this area was the discovery by Fraker et al. (1978) that T-cell dependent responses and thymus atrophy in zinc-deficient mice could be reversed by zinc repletion. Fernandes et al. (1979) drew similar conclusions about the essentiality of zinc for T-cell natural killer function. Maturation and proliferative capacity of these cells may be impaired with long term deficiency (James et al., 1987). A reduced response to antigenic challenge was observed in zinc deficient mice infected with a variety of organisms (Salvin and Rabin, 1984). The area of zinc and infection has been reviewed (Sugarman, 1983).

Data from human subjects support the observations in animals relative to a zinc-immunity connection. Golden et al. (1978) reported a response to zinc in immunity of children with protein-energy malnutrition. Allen et al. (1981) documented improved T-lymphocyte function in patients zinc repleted from a severe deficiency. Similarly, Tapazoglou et al. (1985) increased natural killer activity of lymphoctyes from sickle cell disease patients with concomitant zinc deficiency.

Elderly subjects with immune dysfunction respond to zinc supplementation (Duchateau et al., 1981). In a detailed study, where the zinc status of an elderly population was low (90% below the RDA), Bogden et al. (1987) observed reduced zinc concentrations in mononuclear and polynuclear leukocytes and depressed mitogen responses. These data suggest zinc supplementation is needed to reverse the effects. It must be emphasized of course that in animal studies very high dietary intakes of zinc depress certain aspects of humonal immunity (Mulhern et al., 1985). Depression did not occur at moderate levels (Salvin et al., 1987). This emphasises that any supplementation program must be approached on an experimental basis before widely applied.

The production of sufficient activated T-cells requires interleukin-1 stimulation of resting T-cells and subsequent interleukin-2 production (Dinarello and Mier, 1987). Evidence from studies with old mice suggest that aging produces a decrease in interleukin-1 release from macrophages and a decrease of interleukin-2 production by activated T-cells (Bruley-Rosset and Vergnon, 1984). Kaplan et al.(1988) have showed that human subjects with low zinc status exhibit reduced cellular interleukin-2 production. Interesting in vitro experiments by Winchurch et al.(1987) have shown that thymocytes produced more interleukin-1 when zinc supplemented. Furthermore, Zn^{2+} increased interleukin-4 (B-cell stimulating factor-1) production by T-cells. In the same context, it is of interest that the natural killer activity of lymphocytes from AIDS patients as stimulated in vitro by alpha-interferon can be potentiated through addition of zinc (Cunningham-Rundles, 1984). Stimulation of T-cells by zinc has been related to a zinc-containing ca 0.9 kDa polypeptide termed thymulin (Bach et al., 1988). It has been proposed that thymic hormone production, by whatever means, declines with age and may in this way explain the relationship between zinc and immune dysfunction in the elderly (Dardenne et al.,1988).

Cytokines as a defined series of mediators have a diversity of biologic actions (Dinarello and Mier, 1987). Interleukin-1 has the widest range of activities including the ability to depress acutely serum zinc and iron concentrations in a fashion comparable to endotoxin (DiSilvestro and Cousins, 1984). This response is related in part to induced synthesis of metallothionein. This small 6.5 kDa metalloprotein has been related to the intra cellular metabolism and function of zinc and copper (reviewed in Cousins, 1985; Dunn et al.,1987). Recently, we demonstrated that expression of the metallothionein gene was enhanced in liver, bone marrow and thymus of rats given human recombinant interleukin-1α (Cousins and Leinart, 1988). Coupled with expression is a redistribution of systemic zinc to these three tissues. Zinc is required for many cellular functions including stabilization of membranes, RNA polymerases and "zinc-fingers" of transcription factors (reviewed in Hambidge, 1986). The redistribution has been suggested as a reflection of metabolic prioritization for critical cellular needs for zinc. It is of interest with respect to the metabolic redistribution of zinc that occurs in response to interleukin-1 and some hormones, that with time detailed kinetic analysis shows a release of hepatic zinc to the plasma as $alpha_2$-macroglobulin rather than albumin (Dunn and Cousins, 1988).

The other major role that has been proposed for zinc is related to antioxidant effects. A variety of studies with marginal or deficient zinc intake have demonstrated peroxidation of tissue lipids (Chvapil et al., 1973; Sullivan et al., 1980; Burke and Fenton, 1985; Dreosti and Patrick, 1987). Conversely, high zinc diets may inhibit lipid peroxidation. These phenomena fit the theoretical framework of a functional role for zinc in membrane stabilization (Bettger and O'Dell, 1981). Coppen and Cousins (1988) found that induced free radical formation in cultured rat hepatocytes could be suppressed by addition of zinc to the medium. The effect was observed regardless of whether peroxidative damage was induced by iron or organic oxidants that form free radicals. Zinc increased glutathione peroxidase activity and reduced NADPH-cytochrome c reductase activity. The latter effect of zinc has been reported in vitro with hepatic microsomes (Chvapil et al., 1975; Jeffery, 1983). Zinc also induced metallothionein in the hepatocyte cultures in direct proportion to suppression of free radical production. Metallothionein has been proposed to function as a free radical scavenger (Thornalley and Vasak, 1985; Thomas et al., 1986). Its induction in rats is correlated with protection against ionizing radiation (Matsubara et al., 1987).

The relationship of the antioxidant function for zinc is not clear. However, hormonal regulation of its metabolism suggests that zinc is being deposited to sites of host defense activity. The relationship of this role to zinc nutrition in the elderly is uncertain, but this nutrient appears to have properties that may protect against degenerative disease.

CONCLUSION

The purpose of this brief review has been to highlight certain aspects of host defense roles of copper, iron, selenium and zinc as they could relate to the elderly. It is of concern that with advancing age, we are at a point in the life cycle when these nutrients may be in the most limited supply. Therefore, it is ironic that functional needs of these nutrients at the cellular level on a precise cellular basis may be the most critical. Further, research needs must relate to clearly defining exact functions of these nutrients and the value to adequate nutritional status or supplementation in the elderly.

REFERENCES

Aldred AR, Grimes A, Schreiber G, Mercer JF (1987). Rat ceruloplasmin. J Biol Chem 262:2875-2878.

Allen JI, Kay NE, McClain CJ (1981). Severe zinc deficiency in humans: Association with a reversible T-lymphocyte dysfunction. Annals Intern Med 95:154-157.

Aust SD, Morehouse LA, Thomas CE (1985). Role of metals in oxygen radical reactions. J Free Radicals Biol Med 1:3-25.

Bach J-F, Pleau J-M, Savino W, Laussac J-P, Cung M-T, Lefrancier P, Dardenne M (1988). The role of zinc in the biological activity of thymulin, a thymic metallopeptide hormone. In Prasad AS (ed): "Essential and Toxic Trace Elements in Human Health and Disease," New York: Alan R. Liss, Inc, pp 319-328.

Barber EF, Cousins RJ (1988). Interleukin-1-stimulated induction of ceruloplasmin synthesis in normal and copper-deficient rats. J Nutr 118:375-381.

Bettger WJ, O'Dell BL (1981). A critical physiological role of zinc in the structure and function of biomembranes. Life Sci 28:1425-1438.

Blumberg JB, Meydani SN (1986). Role of dietary antioxidants in aging. In Hutchinson ML, Munro, HN (eds): "Nutrition and Aging," Orlando FL: Academic Press, pp 85-97.

Bogden JD, Oleske JM, Munves EM, Lavenhar MA, Bruening KS, Kemp FW, Holding KJ, Denny TN Louria DB (1987). Zinc and immunocompetence in the elderly: baseline data on zinc nutriture and immunity in unsupplemented subjects. Am J Clin Nutr 46:101-109.

Bruley-Rosset M, Vergnon I (1984). Interleukin-1 synthesis and activity in aged mice. Mech Age Devel 24:247-264.

Burk RF (1986). Selenium and cancer: Meaning of serum selenium levels. J Nutr 116:1584-1586.

Burke JP, Fenton MR (1985). Effect of a zinc-deficient diet on lipid peroxidation in liver and tumor subcellular membranes. Proc Soc Exp Biol Med 179:187-191.

Cerutti PA (1985). Prooxidant states and tumor promotion. Science 227:375-381.

Chandra RK (1988). Trace element regulation of immunity and infection: Quantitative considerations for optimum immunity. In Prasad AS (ed): "Essential and Toxic Trace Elements in Human Health and Disease," New York: Alan R. Liss, Inc, pp 337-346.

Chvapil M, Ryan JN, Elias SL, Peng YM (1973). Protective effect of zinc on carbon tetrachloride-induced liver injury in rats. Exp Molec Pathol 19:186-196.

Chvapil M, Ludwig JC, Sipes IG, Misiorowski RL (1975). Inhibition of NADPH oxidation and related drug oxidation in liver microsomes by zinc. Biochem Pharmacol 25:1787-1791.

Chow CK, Tappel AL (1974). Response to glutathione peroxidase to dietary selenium in rats. J Nutr 104:444-451.

Coppen D, Cousins RJ (1987). Zinc suppression of free radicals induced in cultures of rat hepatocytes by iron, t-butyl hydroperoxide and 3-methyl indole. Proc Soc Exp Biol Med -- submitted.

Crapo JD, Tierney DF (1974). Superoxide dismutase and pulmonary oxygen toxicity. Amer J Physiol 226:6.

Cousins RJ (1985). Absorption, transport, and hepatic metabolism of copper and zinc: Special reference to metallothionein and ceruloplasmin. Physiol Rev 65:238-309.

Cousins RJ, Leinart AS (1988). Tissue specific regulation of zinc metabolism and metallothionein genes by interleukin-1. FASEB J -- in press.

Cunningham-Rundles S (1984). Nutritional factors in immune response. In White PL, Selvey N (eds): "Malnutrition: Determinants and Consequences," New York: Alan R. Liss, Inc, pp 233-244.

Cutler RG (1985). Peroxide-producing potential of tissues: Inverse correlation with longevity of mammalian species. Proc Natl Acad Sci 82:4798-4802.

Dardenne M, Wade S, Savino W, Nabarra B, Prasad AS, Bach J-F (1988). Thymulin and zinc deficiency. In Prasad AS (ed): "Essential and Toxic Trace Elements in Human Health and Disease," New York: Alan R. Liss, Inc, pp 329-336.

Dinarello CA (1987). Biology of interleukin 1. FASEB J 2:108-115.

Dinarello CA, Meir JW (1987). Lymphokines. New Eng J Med 317:940-945.

DiSilvestro RA, Cousins RJ (1984). Mediation of endotoxin-induced changes in zinc metabolism in rats. Am J Physiol 247:E436–E441.

DiSilvestro RA, David, EA (1986). Enzyme immunoassay for ceruloplasmin: application to cancer patient serum. Clinica Chimica Acta 158:287–292.

DiSilvestro RA, Barber EF, David EA, Cousins RJ (1988). An enzyme-linked immunoabsorbent assay for rat ceruloplasmin. Biol Trace Elem Res 15:In Press.

Dreosti IE, Patrick EJ (1987). Zinc, ethanol, and lipid peroxidation in adult and fetal rats. Biol Trace Elem Res 14:179–191.

Duchateau J, Delepesse G, Vrijens R, Collet H (1981). Beneficial effects of oral zinc supplementation on the immune response of old people. Amer J Med 70:1001–1004.

Dunn MA, Blalock TL, Cousins RJ (1987). Metallothionein. Proc Soc Exp Biol Med 185:107–119.

Dunn MA, Cousins RJ (1988). Kinetics and modeling of zinc metabolism in the rat: Effects of dibutyryl cyclic AMP. FASEB J 2:A634.

Fields M, Ferretti RJ, Smith JC, Reiser S (1984). Interaction between dietary carbohydrate and copper nutriture on lipid peroxidation in rat tissues. Biol Trace Elem Res 6:379–390.

Fraker PJ, DePasquale-Jardieu P, Zwickl CM, Luecke RW (1978). Regeneration of T-cell helper function in zinc-deficient adult mice. Proc Natl Acad Sci 75:5660–5664.

Fraker PJ, Gershwin ME, Good RA, Prasad A (1986). Interrelationships between zinc and immune function. Fed Proc 45:1474–1479.

Fernandes G, Nair M, Onoe K, Tanaka T, Floyd R, Good RA (1979). Impairment of cell-mediated immunity functions by dietary zinc deficiency in mice. Proc Natl Acad Sci 76:457–461.

Frieden E (1986). Perspectives on copper biochemistry. Clin Physiol Biochem 4:11–19.

Garfinkel D (1986). Is aging inevitable? The intracellular zinc deficiency hypothesis of aging. Med Hypoth 19:117–137.

Goldblum SE, Cohen DA, Jay M, McClain CJ (1987). Interleukin 1-induced depression of iron and zinc: role of granulocytes and lactoferrin. Am J Physiol 252:E27–32.

Golden MNH, Golden BE, Harland PSEG, Jackson AA (1978). Zinc and immunocompetence in protein-energy malnutrition. Lancet 2:1226-1227.

Halliwell B (1987). Oxidants and human disease: some new concepts. FASEB J 1:358-364.

Hambidge KM, Casey CE, Krebs NF (1986). Zinc. In Mertz W (ed): "Trace Elements in Human and Animal Nutrition, Vol 2," Orlando, FL: Academic Press, Inc, pp 1-137.

Hentze MW, Caughman SW, Rouault TA, Barriocanal JG, Dancis A, Harford JB, Klausner RD (1987). Identification of the iron-responsive element for the translational regulation of human ferritin mRNA. Science 238:1570-1573.

Heresi G (1986). Trace elements and immunity. In Taylor TG, Jenkins NK (eds): "Proceedings 13th Internat Cong of Nutr," London: John Libbey Co, pp 729-733.

Idzerda RL, Huebers H, Finch CA, McKnight GS (1986). Rat transferrin gene expression: Tissue-specific regulation by iron deficiency. Proc Natl Acad Sci 83:3723-3727.

Ip C (1985). Selenium inhibition of chemical carcinogenesis. Fed Proc 44:2573-2578.

James SJ, Swendseid M, Makinodan T (1987). Macrophage-mediated depression of T-cell proliferation in zinc-deficient mice. J Nutr 117:1982-1988.

Jeffery EH (1983). The effect of zinc on NADPH oxidation and monooxygenase activity in rat hepatic microsomes. Cell Pharmacol 23:467-473.

Kaplan J, Hess JW, Prasad AS (1988). Impairment of immune function in the elderly: Association with mild zinc deficiency. In Prasad AS (ed): "Essential and Toxic Trace Elements in Human Health and Disease," New York: Alan R. Liss, Inc, pp 309-317.

Koschinsky ML, Funk WD, Van Oost BA, MacGillivray RTA (1986). Complete cDNA sequence of human preceruloplasmin. Proc Natl Acad Sci 83:5086-5090.

Kubow S, Bray TM, Bettger WJ (1986). Effects of dietary zinc and copper on free radical production in rat lung and liver. Can J Physiol Pharmacol 64:1281-1285.

Lawrence RA, Jenkinson SG (1987). Effects of copper deficiency on carbon tetrachloride-induced lipid peroxidation. J Lab Clin Med 109:134-140.

LeBoeuf RA, Hoekstra WG (1985). Changes in cellular glutathione levels: possible relation to selenium-mediated anticarcinogenesis. Fed Proc 44:2563-2567.

Levander OA (1987). A global view of human selenium nutrition. Ann Rev Nutr 7:227-250.

Matsubara J, Tajima Y, Karasawa M (1987). Metallothionein induction as a potent means of radiation protection in mice. Rad Res 111:267-275.

Milner JA (1985). Effect of selenium on virally induced and transplantable tumor models. Fed Proc 44:2568-2572.

Mulhern SA, Vessey AR, Taylor GL, Magruder LE (1985). Suppression of antibody response by excess dietary zinc exposure during certain stages of ontogeny. Proc Soc Exp Biol Med 180:453-461.

Newman S, Guzelian PS (1982). Stimulation of de novo synthesis of cytochrome P-450 by phenobarbital in primary nonproliferating cultures of adult rat hepatocytes. Proc Nat Acad Sci 79:2922-2926.

Prohaska JR, Lukasewycz OA (1981). Copper deficiency suppresses the immune response of mice. Science 213:559-561.

Prohaska JR, Downing SW, Lukasewycz OA (1983). Chronic dietary copper deficiency alters biochemical and morphological properties of mouse lymphoid tissues. J Nutr 113:1583-1590.

Rotruck J, Pope A, Ganther H, Swanson A, Hafeman D, Hoekstra W (1973). Selenium: Biochemical role as a component of glutathione peroxidase. Science 179:588-590.

Salvin SB, Rabin BS (1984). Resistance and susceptibility to infection in inbred murine strains. Cell Immunol 87:546-552.

Salvin SB, Horecker BL, Pan L-X, Rabin BS (1987). The effect of dietary zinc and prothymosin α on cellular immune responses of RF/J mice. Clin Immunol Immunopathol 43:281-288.

Serfass RE, Ganther HE (1975). Defective microbicidal activity in glutathione peroxidase-deficient neutrophils of selenium-deficient rats. Nature(London) 255:640-641

Serfass RE, Ganther HE (1976). Effects of dietary selenium and tocopherol on glutathione peroxidase and superoxide dismutase activities in rat phagocytes. Life Sci 19:1139-1144.

Stocker R, Ames BN (1987). Potential role of conjugated bilirubin and copper in the metabolism of lipid peroxides in bile. Proc Natl Acad Sci 84:8130-8134.

Sugarman B, (1983). Zinc and infection. Rev Infect Dis 5:137-147.

Sullivan JF, Jetton MM, Hahn HJK, Burch RE (1980). Enhanced lipid peroxidation in liver microsomes of zinc deficient rats. Am J Clin Nutr 110:51-56.

Tapazoglou E, Prasad AS, Hill G, Brewer GJ, Kaplan J (1985). Decreased natural killer cell activity in patients with zinc deficiency with sickle cell disease. J Lab Clin Med 105:19-22.

Thomas JP, Bachowski GJ, Girotti AW (1986). Inhibition of cell membrane lipid peroxidation by cadmium- and zinc-metallothioneins. Biochim Biophys Acta 884:448-461.

Thornalley PJ, Vasak M (1985). Possible role for metallothionein in protection against radiation-induced oxidative stress. Kinetics and mechanism of its reaction with superoxide and hydroxyl radicals. Biochem Biophys Acta 827:36-44.

Weinberg ED (1986). Iron, infection, and neoplasia. Clin Physiol Biochem 4:50-60.

Winchurch RA, Togo J, Adler WH (1987). Supplemental zinc (Zn^{2+}) restores antibody formation in cultures of aged spleen cells II. Effects on mediator production. Eur J Immunol 17:127-132.

Zahringer J, Baliga BS, Munro HN (1976). Novel mechanism for translational control in regulation of ferritin synthesis by iron. Proc Nat Acad Sci 73:857-861.

Mineral Homeostasis in the Elderly, pages 223–244
© 1989 Alan R. Liss, Inc.

NUTRITIONAL DEFICITS IN THE CHRONICALLY ILL ELDERLY

William P. Steffee, M.D.,Ph.D.

J. Carlos Teran, M.D.

Saint Vincent Charity Hospital
Cleveland, Ohio 44115

Perhaps the best way to introduce the discussion of trace element requirements relative to the nutritional status of chronically ill hospitalized elderly is to say that after 15 years of treating an overabundance of elderly in the hospital setting, I clearly do not know what I am doing relative to trace element nutrition. I am pleased to be able to review what is known relative to nutritional aspects in this particular population, since I believe that this perspective represents the state of the art in the field at this time.

From an even broader nutritional perspective, there are several questions relative to the hospitalized, older patient. Are the chronically ill elderly malnourished, or simply old and/or sick? Are there identifiable perturbations and micronutrient nutrition in the chronically ill elderly? How and where can we assess nutritional status of this particular group of individuals? Can we intervene nutritionally? Should we intervene nutritionally: does nutrition intervention make any difference at all in clinical outcome?

Are the chronically ill elderly malnourished? They probably are. The reasons for malnutrition in the elderly are legion and have been discussed

many times. They are worth reciting. There has
been a general deterioration of the "normal" diet
at large in the population. Where as the concept
of the attainment of 4 food groups in 3 square
meals/day is laudable, it is undoubtedly true that
in many instances the elderly patient does not
gain access to a broad spectrum of food on a
consistent basis. Recent difficulties in
defining a consensus relative to the definition of
the Recommended Daily Allowances for the
population at large is confounded to even a
greater extent if one specifically explores
requirements of a chronically ill elderly
population.

There are many socio/economic issues
impacting on the elderly's ability to attain
proper nourishment;inadequate income, death of a
close family member, social/economic "abandonment"
by the family, and many others outside the point
of this presentation.

Chronic diseases such as cardiac cachexia and
bowel atrophy from many different causes induce
conditions which create impairments from a
social/functional perspective. Many of these
diseases create anorexia and a decreased desire to
attain food, which can predispose the elderly
patient to nutritional inadequacies.
Atherosclerosis in all of its clinical
presentations, whether it be heart disease, stroke
or dementia, has a major propensity to decrease
the elderly patient's ability to acquire and/or
absorb nutrients. Diabetes Mellitus and all of
its complications induces abnormalities in
nutritional status. Cancer induces anorexia and
weight loss. When neoplasms involve the
gastrointestinal tract, the potential obstructive
nature of the disease compounds nutritional
inadequacies. When therapy is instituted, whether
chemotherapy, radiation therapy or surgery,
nutritional status again plummets in most all
cases. Dementia from whatever etiology whether
Alzheimer's disease or dementia related to other
medical disorders, impairs both patient's judgment

relative to diet and ultimately, the ability to consume food in any manner what so ever.

Drug nutrient interactions abound and interfere either directly with the person's ability to eat (such as digitalis creating nausea and loss of appetite) or indirectly due to endogenous drug nutrient interactions.

Identifiable perturbations in micronutrient nutrition are expressed in the elderly population. For the past several years the Nutrition Intervention Team at Saint Vincent Charity Hospital and Health Center in Cleveland has been measuring serum copper and zinc levels in patients consulted to the nutrition support service. Our experience reflects that of others, whereby blood levels become uninterpretable due to the influence of other diseases, complications and/or therapy. Does low levels reflect deficiency or redistribution? It would be most appropriate to review the current status of our knowledge relative to the more common trace elements found in the clinical setting particularly, as they are reflected in the various disease states to which the elderly are exposed.

It is important to explain that our search was restricted to blood samples because they are the only source easily available in clinical practice without an invasive procedure. There is increasing evidence that in many instances blood levels of trace elements do not correlate with the whole body levels because of redistribution changes between blood and tissues. The finding of an altered blood level does not necessarily imply the need of treatment for such condition and conversely a normal blood level in the presence of deficiency signs should prompt substitution. Until we develop a reliable bedside test to estimate whole-body trace element levels we will have to rely in blood levels, but caution is suggested in the interpretation of such results before deciding to treat.

Zinc

Zinc is the most widely studied of the trace
elements. Zinc blood levels have been studied in
many diseases and zinc deficiency has been well
characterized. A great number of clinical trials
have studied the effect of zinc supplementation in
the treatment of deficiency signs such as leg
ulcers, hypogonadism, taste alterations, etc.

Short term starvation has been shown to
transiently increase zinc blood levels (Elia, et
al.,1984.; Tulikoura, et al.,1986.; Henry, et
al.,1975.). Zinc levels return to normal or
decrease after a few days and with renutrition.
These changes are believed to be due to
redistribution. Urine zinc excretion also
increases during the first days of acute
starvation and then returns to normal probably
reflecting an increase of the zinc delivered to
the kidneys (Elia, et al.,1984.).

Many investigators consistently report a
decrease on blood zinc levels in uremia (Abu-
Homdam, et al.,1986.; Beerbower, et al.,1985.;
Condon, et al.,1970.; Monsouri, et al.,1970.;
Halsted, et al.,1970.; Mahajan, et al.,1982.;
Tsukamoto, et al.,1980.; Lindeman, et al.,1978.).
The mechanism of this alteration is not well
understood but may involve a decrease in intake
or a decrease in absorption or bioavailability of
zinc (Abu-Homdam, et al.,1986.). Dialysis and
renal transplantation has been reported to
normalize plasma zinc levels (Beerbower, et
al.,1985.; Monsouri, et al.1970.; Mahajan, et
al.1983.). Although there are reports of
improvement of the taste disturbances and of the
hypogonadism associated with uremia by zinc
supplementation (Mahajan, et al.,1982.), other
authors suggest a redistribution phenomenon
(Condon, et al.,1970).

Plasma zinc has been repeatedly noted to be
low in both alcoholic and non-alcoholic advanced
liver diseases such as hepatitis or cirrhosis

(Halsted, et al.,1970.; Lindeman, et al.,1978.; Valberg, et al.,1985.; Halsted, et al.,1968.; Sullivan, et al.,1970.; Versieck, et al.,1974.). The mechanism is probably the loss of the renal threshold for zinc resulting in elevated urinary zinc concentrations (Halsted, et al.,1968.; Sullivan, et al.,1970.). Plasma albumin levels do not correlate with zinc levels so low plasma zinc levels are not supposed to be due to a decrease in the plasma protein fixation (Lindeman, et al.,1978.). In alcoholic liver disease, a component of zinc malabsorption has been reported which is believed to be produced by a direct effect of alcohol on the intestinal mucosa (Valberg, et al.,1985.). Some investigators believe that the hypogonadism observed in cirrhosis could be related to zinc deficiency (Sullivan, et al.,1970.).

Most work relating zinc levels and cardiac disease has been done in acute myocardial infarction (Halsted, et al.,1970.; Lindeman, et al.,1972.; McBean, et al.,1974.). In this disease the decrease of blood zinc is transient and returns to normal after the acute phase, suggesting a redistribution phenomenon. More work needs to be done to characterize the changes of zinc in other cardiac diseases and in chronic cardiac failure.

Extensive intestinal diseases such as Crohn's disease, the short gut syndrome, and also pancreatic exocrine insufficiency, alone or associated with cystic fibrosis have all been reported to cause zinc deficiency (Halsted, et al.,1970.; McHain, et al.,1983.; Faber, et al.,1978.; Fabris, et al.,1985.). Growth retardation, a known complication of cystic fibrosis and untreated Crohn's disease, could be related to zinc deficiency (Halsted, et al.,1970.; Mchain, et al.,1983.). In all these diseases, urinary zinc is low and they are believed to represent true depletion states and not redistribution phenomena.

Major surgical procedures consistently induce a drop in plasma zinc levels (Lindeman, et al.,1972.; Tengrup, et al.,1977.; Hallbook, et al.,1977.; Myers, et al.,1984.; Fawaz, et al.,1985.). Urinary zinc has been observed to increase in some reports (Lindeman, et al.,1972.) suggesting a true loss of body zinc but others suggest that the transient plasma zinc decrease is due to redistribution (Hallbook, et al.,1977.). Minor operations, such as herniorraphy, have no effect on plasma zinc levels (Tengrup, et al.,1977.). As the role of zinc in tissue repair is well established, zinc deficiency should be considered in postoperative patients with wound dehiscence or chronic ulcers (Fawaz, et al.,1985).

Extensive burns produce a drop in blood zinc levels that might last two weeks (Boosalis, et al.,1988.; Cohen, et al.,1973.). Some authors have proposed that this is an acute phase reaction to stress, suggesting a redistribution mechanism (Boosalis, et al.,1988.), but others have reported an increase of urinary zinc and hypogeusia suggesting a true deficiency state (Cohen, et al.,1973.). The same pattern has been described in head trauma patients (McClain, et al.,1986.), whether supplementary zinc should be given to these patients is not well established (Boosalis, et al.,1988.).

Acute and chronic infections also lower plasma zinc levels (Halsted, et al.,1970.; Lindeman, et al.,1972.). Low zinc levels last until infection is controlled (Lindeman, et al.,1972.). This could represent an acute redistribution phenomenon, but if prolonged, could interfere with immune response. Pulmonary infections, (the old man's friend) especially active tuberculosis, are among the most consistent causes of low plasma zinc levels (Halsted, et al.,1970.).

Diabetic patients have a higher than normal incidence of low blood zinc levels (McClain, et al.,1986.; Kumar, et al.,1974.; Kinlaw, et al.,1983.), even though some studies do not confirm this finding (Chooi, et al.,1976.). Excessive urinary zinc losses are well documented in this group, and are more important if proteinuria is present (McClain, et al.,1986.). Also, defective absorption of zinc in the intestine has been proposed (McClain, et al.,1986.). This finding is of particular interest due to the known role of zinc in pancreatic insulin secretion. In thyroid disease, plasma zinc has been reported as normal, although an inverse correlation of the thyroid hormone levels and erythrocyte zinc was present (Aihara, et al.,1984.).

Several neoplastic diseases such as lung cancer, carcinoma of the esophagus, other digestive carcinomas, sarcoma, and chronic lymphocytic leukemia, have been reported to reduce blood zinc levels (Issell, et al.,1981.; Morgan, et al.,1970.; Mellow, et al.,1983.; Inutsuka, et al.,1978.; Fisher, et al.,1976.; Beguin, et al.,1987.; Davies, et al.,1968.). Bronchogenic carcinomas are known for inducing the most striking decreases in plasma zinc levels (Davies, et al.,1968.). Some of the manifestations of cancer like anorexia, taste loss and immune impairment could benefit from zinc supplementation. Interestingly, depressed red blood cell zinc levels but not plasma levels have been proposed as a marker of metastatic spread (Gorodetsky, et al.,1985.).

Controversy exists about whether old age per se causes zinc deficiency or this is always secondary to underlying diseases (Gershwin, et al.,1987.; Murphy, et al.,1985.; Davies, et al.,1968.). Some studies report a tendency towards low zinc levels in healthy elderly and a decrease in zinc intake has been demonstrated in this age group (Hsu, et al.,1979.; Chooi, et al.,1976.). It also could be that a different normal range for blood zinc levels should be used for geriatric patients. The high incidence of taste and appetite alterations among the elderly due to the normal aging process should be considered before promoting zinc supplementation.

Copper

Copper is the second most well studied trace element in clinical medicine. Serum values are difficult to interpret due to redistribution changes and should not be used as a guide for copper requirements (Shike, et al.,1981.). Most of the cases of copper deficiency reported are children and are beyond the scope of this review, but in certain diseases true copper deficiency can develop in adults (Solomons, et al.,1985.). Another confounding factor is the fact that blood copper levels tend to rise with any disease that induces cholestasis or inflammation thus being able to mask underlying deficiency states.

Acute and chronic malnutrition induces a drop in blood copper levels in children (Solomons, et al.,1985.) but this has not been well explored in adults. Most of the work related to copper in starvation in adults includes patients with catabolic disease or with patients receiving total parenteral nutrition, so it is difficult to isolate the effect of starvation alone in blood copper levels (Tulikoura, et al.,1986.; Shike, et al.,1981.). It appears that it takes long periods of starvation to induce copper deficiency, if there are no abnormal losses, and that the content of copper as a contaminant in drinking water is enough to fulfill the requirements.

In studies of copper blood levels in uremia the results range from normal (Monsouri, et al.,1970.) to high (Tsukamoto, et al.,1980.). The last study included 55 non dialyzed patients whereas the first study only included 15 patients. More work is needed to solve these apparently contradictory results.

In all diseases that induce cholestasis, such as hepatitis cirrhosis (Versieck, et al.,1974.) or obstructive jaundice, copper has consistently been elevated in blood. This is consistent with the knowledge that bile is the main route of copper excretion. Whether copper should be restricted in these conditions to prevent toxicity remains to be established.

Although balance studies in patients with increased intestinal losses such as malabsorption and fistula, have consistently demonstrated an increase in requirements (Shike, et al.,1981.; Bozzetti, et al.,1983.), it appears that the normal blood copper levels found in these patients do not reflect the whole body copper status (Shike, et al.,1981.). In patients with jejunoileal bypass surgery for morbid obesity, serum copper levels have been reported as lower than normal (Faber, et al.,1978.).

An increase in plasma copper has consistently been reported in the first postoperative days in different types of surgery (Myers, et al.,1984.; Bozzetti, et al.,1983.; Hallbook, et al.,1980.). This is believed to be due to a rise in ceruloplasmin as an acute phase reactant (Myers, et al.,1984.). In a more detailed study this has been shown to consist of a two phase process, with a drop in the first hours followed by a rise that remains for several days (Myers, et al.,1984.).

Acute injuries and burns show an acute phase response with an elevation of copper and ceruloplasmin levels in the following few days (Solomons, et al.,1985.; Boosalis, et al.,1986.). Increase in urinary copper losses could induce copper depletion in severe trauma and burns (Solomons, et al.,1985.).

Bacterial, parasite and mycobacterial infections induce an increase in blood copper levels as with any other inflammatory condition (Solomons, et al.,1985). To our knowledge no work has been done in critically ill septicemic patients as a guideline for nutritional support.

High blood copper levels have been reported
in many different neoplastic diseases as multiple
myeloma (Goodman, et al.,1967.), leukemia (Beguin,
et al.,1987.; Hrgovcic, et al.,1968.), non-Hodgkin
lymphoma (Cohen, et al.,1983.; Sham, et al.,1983.;
Shah-Reddy, et al.,1980.; Roguljic, et al.,1980.;
Hrgovcic, et al.,1968.; Hrgovicic, et al.,1973.),
Hodgkin disease (Hrgovcic, et al.,1973.), hepatic
carcinoma (Miattoo, et al.,1985.), melanoma
(Fisher, et al.,1981.), sarcoma (Fisher, et
al.,1976.; Breiter, et al.,1978.), digestive
carcinomas (Inutsuka, et al.,1978.), metastatic
carcinomas (Gorodetsky, et al.,1985.), and
colorectal carcinoma (Putzki, et al.,1985.).
Elevation of copper blood levels has been shown to
correlate with the extension of the disease in non
Hodgkin lymphomas and Hodgkin disease. Whether
this phenomenon can camouflage total body copper
deficiency in some cancers, particularly in
digestive cancer, has not been established.

Serum copper concentration is increased in
atherosclerosis, both coronary and cerebral, and
in hypertension (Hsu, et al.,1979.). Diabetes
Mellitus can be associated to true copper
deficiency and low blood copper levels apparently
due to copper losses in urine (Hsu, et al.,1979.).
Hyperthyroidism has been shown to raise blood
copper concentration (Aihara, et al.,1984.).

Blood copper levels have been found to be
normal in geriatric populations with no disease
(Gershwin, et al.,1987.; Murphy, et al.,1985.),
but other investigators report a tendency of blood
copper levels to rise with age (Hsu, et al.,1979).

Selenium

Selenium has also been studied in clinical
setting but some gaps in the present knowledge are
still apparent. Most of the work has been devoted
to selenium deficiency as a predisposing factor
for neoplasia but this could be considered a
result rather than a cause of low selenium blood
levels.

The effects of acute and chronic starvation on blood selenium levels still need to be studied. It is reported that long term starvation can cause selenium depletion particularly in regions where selenium content of water and soil is low (Robinson, et al.,1979.).

In patients with chronic renal failure, blood levels have been found to be lower than normal (Miller, et al.,1983.; Kallistratos, et al.,1985.). Dialysis did not appear to normalize blood selenium in one report (Kallistratos, et al.,1985.). It is not well established whether this corresponds to a true deficiency or to a redistribution or dilution effect.

Low blood selenium levels have also been reported in cirrhotics (Miller, et al.,1983.; Johansson, et al.,1986.). Selenium in blood does not always correlate with albumin levels in cirrhosis (Miller, et al.,1983.). Alcoholism alone does not decrease blood selenium (Johansson, et al.,1986.).

Selenium deficiency is a well known rare cause of dilated cardiomyopathy but this is more a consequence than a cause. To our knowledge no work addresses the effect of chronic cardiac failure of any cause on selenium blood levels.

In patients with Crohn's disease blood selenium has been reported to be normal (Shamberger, et al.,1973.). Work still needs to be done to quantify the amount of selenium losses in malabsorption, short bowel syndrome and fistulae.

Selenium levels in blood has been noted to be low in patients with cancer (Anonymous, 1970.) specifically gastrointestinal carcinoma (Shamberger, et al.,1973.; Pothier, et al.,1987.), Hodgkin disease (Miller, et al.,1983.), but not in breast cancer or rectal carcinoma (Shamberger, et al.,1973.). The role of selenium deficiency as a risk factor to neoplasia has been reviewed extensively (Anonymous, 1970.),but a possibility exists that cancer could be a cause of selenium deficiency, particularly in zones of the world with poor selenium intake (Robinson, et al.,1979.). Not enough information is available regarding the effect of trauma, burns, surgery or infections on blood selenium levels. Blood selenium does not decrease with aging (Shamberger, et al.,1973.) but red blood cell selenium has been reported to be low in old patients without a correlation with plasma levels (Miller, et al.,1983.). In selenium deficient regions of the world, the geriatric population has been reported to have a high incidence of low blood selenium (Robinson, et al.,1979.).

Manganese

Information about manganese blood levels in disease is still very incomplete.

A report of the effect of short term starvation on manganese in patients with catabolic diseases showed normal blood levels (Tulikouri, et al.,1986.). Probably as long as trace amounts are ingested in water deficiency is prevented, but in patients on long term total parenteral nutrition deficiency can develop. Low manganese levels have been reported in patients on chronic hemodialysis but this is considered to be an effect of the low manganese concentration in hemodialysate fluid designed to prevent manganese intoxication (Hosokawa, et al.,1987.). Apparently, manganese blood levels are not affected by renal failure per se because urinary losses of manganese are very low (Hosokawa, et al.,1987.). The main route of manganese excretion is the bile. High blood manganese levels have been reported in cirrhosis and hepatitis (Versieck, et al.,1974.).

There is a lack of information about the effect of many diseases on manganese blood levels, for example; in trauma, sepsis, surgery, starvation, malabsorption, chronic failure, diabetes, and cancer. Also, studies are needed regarding manganese status of the geriatric population.

Chromium

Most of the studies of chromium status in disease address the issue of glucose intolerance. Information on other diseases is very scattered.

Chromium deficiency is well known to cause glucose intolerance (Shroeder, et al.,1967.; Anderson, et al.,1986.; Wabilach, et al.,1985.). Chromium blood levels have been reported to be normal in the American diabetic population (Rabinowitz, et al.,1980.), but low in diabetics in England (Morris, et al.,1985.). As the main route of chromium excretion is the urine, it also has been proposed that low chromium blood levels could be the result (and not only the cause) of urinary losses in diabetics (Donaldson, et al.,1981.). This could constitute a vicious cycle in which uncontrolled diabetics loose chromium in urine and become chromium deficient thus aggravating glucose intolerance and polyuria.

Catabolic diseases can increase urinary losses of chromium and eventually lower blood chromium levels (Anderson, et al.,1986.). More information is required about particular diseases but chromium deficiency could contribute to glucose intolerance in long term catabolic patients. A study in a geriatric population showed normal blood chromium levels even though their mean ingestion was below normal (Bunker, et al.,1984.), but other studies show that a significant proportion of the geriatric population improve their glucose tolerance with chromium supplementation (Hsu, et al.,1979.).

There is a lack of information about the effects on chromium blood level of diseases such as cardiac failure, hepatic failure, renal failure, malabsorption, cancer and short term starvation.

How/where can we access nutritional status?
One of the major needs for research in trace
element nutrition in the elderly is simply to
define and identify the appropriate place to
monitor trace element nutrition in this group of
individuals. The normal population, residing at
home and not afflicted with disease would be the
ideal starting point, however, the use of broad
survey techniques to study this population will
probably not add a great deal of insight relative
to our understanding of trace element metabolism
in the chronically ill elderly. Since many
elderly end up their lives in nursing homes, it
might be reasonable to address this population.
However, in many instances nursing homes lack the
resources, both financially and personnel to
seriously address issues of trace element
nutrition.

Patients admitted to the acute care hospital
have nutritional status confounded by their
illnesses, however, the resources are available
for the study of nutritional status in this
particular population. Most hospitals do have
identifiable nutrition support teams in addition
to dietary departments. Recent accreditation
requirements for hospitals have demanded a
nutrition assessment of all patients upon
admission to the hospital setting. It would seem
most appropriate to explore the means by which
these health care providers can gain the knowledge
and the ability to begin to address the assessment
of trace element nutriture in this group of the
population.

Nutritional assessment in the modern hospital
setting demands an assessment of nutritional
history, status, and requirements.

Can We Intervene Nutritionally?

One of the more significantly advances in the
realm of nutrition in recent years has been the
evolution of our ability to intervene
nutritionally in nearly any patient encountered in

the hospital setting. Whereas, an optimum diet consumed by mouth on an voluntary basis is clearly the ultimate goal, for most patients admitted to the hospital that are consulted by the nutrition support team, the inability to eat is the primary issue associated with their disease process. To effectively treat such individuals generally requires the application of nutrition intervention techniques. Enteral hyperalimentation, the provision of all nutrients by feeding tubes is a common event in the hospital setting. Specific formulas have been developed for specific diseases, and even now specific geriatric formulas are being introduced into the market place, and modified to meet what currently we think to be the specific requirements of the elderly subject. In such solutions, trace elements may be modified however, as previously discussed, the precise rationale for these changes can not be clearly stated. Intravenous nutrition, either by the peripheral route or more long term total parenteral nutrition via a central catheter, is now commonplace. Our ability to meet specific trace element requirements of the elderly population by this route is clearly available. We are severely constrained, however, relative to our lack of knowledge as to what to treat, when, and in what amounts.

Should We Intervene Nutritionally In The Elderly Population?

We have gained the ability to intervene for any living human being and meet the nutritional requirements of that individual, even if no intestinal tract exists. There is considerable need to evaluate whether such intervention makes any ultimate difference in clinical outcome, particularly for an elderly individual. One of the most perplexing problems facing clinical nutritionists is to make a decision whether an elderly patient, appearing terminally ill, is in fact truly ill to a degree that might cause death, or simply has been allowed to become so malnourished that the impression of terminal

illness is imposed upon the clinician. If the
individual is dying of an incurable terminal
disease, then clearly we should not apply the
nutritional intervention techniques. If in fact
however, the clinical expression represents a
potentially reversible nutritional defect, then
the techniques available to us should be utilized
to their fullest extent in order to restore health
and functional capacity. It is entirely probable
that a clinical decision is made to allow an
elderly patient to die of the effects of
starvation when in fact, the only defect may be a
severe deficiency or disruption in trace element
metabolism which could be relatively easy reversed
if proper knowledge were made available to the
treating physician.

     Now that we have the capacity to treat any
individual for whom a chance exists for recovery
from any other primary illness that might be
present, we in the clinical arena need and, in
fact, now demand that sufficient trace element
research be conducted to allow us to make proper
decisions relative to the care of these
individuals. We literally do not know what we are
doing from a trace element prospective. The
effects of our lack of knowledge can be far
reaching indeed. It is the hope of many of us,
that research will be performed and directed
towards the clinical setting, particularly the
diseased elderly subject, which will provide us
with the ability to restore health, and
ultimately, to prevent the emergence of
potentially life threatening malnutrition.

REFERENCES:

Abu-Homdam DK, Mahajan SK, et al., (1986). Zinc
    tolerance test in uremia. Ann Intern Med 104:50-
    52.
Aihara K, Nishi Y, Hatano S, et al. (1984). Zinc,
    copper, manganese and selenium metabolism in
    thyroid disease. Am J Clin Nutr 40:26-35.

Anderson RA, (1986). Chromium metabolism and its role in disease processes in man. Clin Physical Biochem 4:31-41.

Anonymous (1970). Selenium and cancer. Nutrition Reviews 28:75-80.

Beerbower KS, Raess BU, (1985). Erythrocyte, plasma, urine and dialysate zinc levels in patients on continuous ambulatory peritoneal dialysis. Am J Clin Nutr 41:697-702.

Beguin Y, Brasseur F, et al., (1987). Observations of serum trace elements in chronic lymphocytic leukemia. Cancer 60:1842-1846.

Boosalis MG, Solem LD, et al., (1988). Serum zinc response in thermal injury. J Am Coll Nutr 7:69-76.

Boosalis MG, McCall JT, et al., (1986). Serum copper and ceruloplasmin levels and urinary copper excretion in thermal injury. Am J Clin Nutr 44:899-906.

Bozzetti F, Inglese MG, et al.,(1983). Hypocupremia in patients receiving total parenteral nutrition. J Parenteral and Enteral Nutr 7:563-566.

Breiter DN, Diasio RB, et al., (1978). Serum copper and zinc measurements in patients with osteogenic sarcoma. Cancer 42:598-602.

Bunker VW, Lawson MS, (1984). The uptake and excretion of chromium by the elderly, Am J Clin Nutr 39:797-802.

Chooi MK, Todd JK, Boyd ND, (1976). Influence of age and sex on plasma zinc levels in normal and diabetic individuals. Nutr Metabol 20:135-142.

Cohen IK, Schechter PJ, Henkin RI, (1973). Hypogeusia, anorexia, and altered zinc metabolism following thermal burn. JAMA 223:914-916.

Cohen Y, Epelbaum R, et al., (1983). The value of serum copper levels in non-Hodgkin's lymphoma. Cancer 296-300.

Condon CJ, Freeman FM, (1970). Zinc metabolism in renal failure. Ann Intern Med 73:531-36.

Davies IJT, Musa M, Dormandy TL, (1968). Measurements of plasma zinc: part I in health and diseases. J Clin Path 21:359-363.

Davies IJT, Musa M, Dormandy TL, (1968).
Measurements of plasma zinc: part II in
malignant disease. Clin Path 21:363-365.

Donaldson DL, Renner OM, (1981). Chromium (III)
metabolism by the kidney. Ann Clin Lab Sci
11:377-385.

Elia M, Crozier C, Neale G, (1984). Mineral
metabolism during short-term starvation in man.
Clin Chim Acta 139:37-45.

Faber J, Randolph JG, Robbins S, et al., (1978).
Zinc and copper status in young patients
following jejunoileal bypass. J Surg Res 24:83-
86.

Fabris C, Farini R, Favero G, et al., (1985).
Copper, zinc, and copper/zinc ratio in chronic
pancreatitis and pancreatic cancer. Clin
Biochem 18:373-375.

Fawaz F, (1985). Zinc deficiency in surgical
patients: a clinical study. Journal of
Parenteral and Enteral Nutrition 9:364-369.

Fisher, GL, Byres VS, Shifrine M, et al., (1976).
Copper and zinc levels in serum from human
patients with sarcomas. Cancer 37:356-363.

Fisher GL, Spitler LE, McNeill KL, et al.,(1981).
Serum copper and zinc levels in melanoma
patients. Cancer 47:1838-1844.

Gershwin ME, Hurley L, (1987). Trace metals and
immune function in the elderly. Comprehensive
Therapy 13:18-23.

Goodman SI, Rodgerson DO, Kauffman J, (1967).
Hypercupremia in a patient with multiple
myeloma. J Lab Clin Med 70:57-62.

Gorodetsky R, Fuks Z, et al., (1985). Correlation
of erythrocyte and plasma levels of zinc,
copper, and iron with evidence of metastatic
spread. Cancer 55:779-787.

Gregoriadis GC, Apostolidis NS, Romanos AN, et
al., (1982). Postoperative changes in serum
copper value. Surg Gynecol Obstet 154:217-221.

Hallbook T, Hedelin H,(1977). Zinc metabolism and
surgical trauma. Br J Surg 64:271-73.

Hallbook T, Hedelin H, (1980). Changes in serum
copper and serum ceruloplasmin concentration
induced by surgical trauma. Acta Chir Scand
146:371-373.

Halsted JA, Smith JC, (1970). Plasma-zinc in
  health and disease. The Lancet 14:322-24.
Halsted JA, Hackley B, Rudzki C, et al., (1968).
  Plasma zinc concentration in liver diseases.
  Gastroenterology 54:1098-1105.
Henry RW, Elmes ME, (1975). Plasma zinc in acute
  starvation. Br Med J 4(5997):625.
Hosokawa S, Nishitani H, (1987). Role of manganese
  in chronic hemodialysis patients. Int J Artif
  Organs 10:14-16.
Hrgovcic M, Tessmer CF, et al., (1968). Serum
  copper levels in lymphoma and leukemia. Cancer
  21:743-755.
Hrgovcic M, Tessmer CF, et al., (1973).
  Significance of serum copper levels in adult
  patients with Hodgkin's disease. Cancer 31:1337-
  1345.
Hrgovcic M, Tessmer CF, et al., (1973). Serum
  copper observations in patients with malignant
  lymphoma. Cancer 32:1512-1524.
Hsu JM, (1979). Current knowledge on zinc, copper
  and chromium in aging. World Rev Nutr Diet
  33:42-69.
Inutsuka S, Araki S, (1978). Plasma copper and
  zinc levels in patients with malignant tumors of
  digestive organs. Cancer 42:626-631.
Issell BF, MacFadyen BV, (1981). Serum zinc levels
  in lung cancer patients. Cancer 47:1845-1848.
Johansson U, Johansson F, et al., (1986). Selenium
  status in patients with liver cirrhosis and
  alcoholism. Br J Nutr 55:227-233.
Kallistratos G, Evangelou A, et al., (1985).
  Selenium and hemodialysis: serum selenium levels
  in healthy persons, non-cancer and cancer
  patients with chronic renal failure. Nephron
  41:217-222.
Kinlaw WB, Levine AS, et al., (1983). Abnormal
  zinc metabolism in type II diabetes mellitus.
  Am J Med 75:273-277.
Kumar S, Jaya-Rao KS, (1974). Blood and urinary
  zinc levels in diabetes mellitus. Nutr Metabol
  17:231-235.
Lindeman R, Baxter DJ, Yunice AA, et al., (1978).
  Serum concentrations and urinary excretions of

zinc in cirrhosis, nephrotic syndrome and renal insufficiency. Am J Med Sci 275:17-31.

Lindeman RD, Bottomley RG, Cornelison RL, et al., (1972). Influence of acute tissue injury on zinc metabolism in man. J Lab Clin Med 79:452-460.

Mahajan SK, Prasad AS, et al., (1982). Zinc deficiency: a reversible complication of uremia. Am J Clin Nutr 36:1147-11883.

Mahajan S, Abraham J, Hessburg T, et al., (1983). Zinc metabolism and taste acuity in renal transplant recipients. Kid Int 24:Suppl 16: S-310-14.

McBean LD, Smith JC, Berne BH, et al., (1974). Serum zinc and alpha$_2$ - macroglobulin concentration in myocardial infarction, decubitus ulcer, multiple myeloma, prostatic carcinoma, down's syndrome and nephrotic syndrome. Clin Chim Acta 50:43-51.

McClain CJ, Twymon DL, et al., (1986). Serum and urine zinc response in head-injured patients. J Neurosurg 64:224-230.

McHain CJ, Sy L, Gilbert H, et al., (1983). Zinc deficiency - induced retinal dysfunction in Crohn's disease. Dig Dis Sci 28:85-87.

Mellow MH, Layne EA, et al., (1983). Plasma zinc and vitamin A in human squamous carcinoma of the esophagus. Cancer 51:1615-1620.

Miattoo, Casaril M, et al., (1985). Diagnostic and prognostic value of serum copper and plasma dibrinogen in hepatic carcinoma. Cancer 53:774-778.

Miller L, Mills BJ, Blotcky DJ, et al., (1983). Red blood cell and serum selenium concentrations as influenced by age and selected diseases. J Am Coll Nutr 4:331-341.

Monsouri K, Halsted JA, Gombos EA, (1970). Zinc, copper, magnesium and calcium in dialyzed and nondialyzed uremic patient. Arch Intern Med 125:88-93.

Morgan JM, (1970). Cadmium and zinc abnormalities in bronchogenic carcinoma. Cancer 25:1394-1398.

Morris BW, Kemp GJ, Hardisty CA, (1985). Plasma chromium and chromium excretion in diabetes. Clin Chem 31:334-335.

Murphy P, Wadiwale I, Sharland DE, et al., (1985).
  Copper and zinc levels in "healthy" and "sick"
  elderly. J Am Geriatr Soc 33:847-849.
Myers MA, Flick A, et al., (1984). Early plasma
  protein and mineral changes after surgery: a two
  stage process. J Clin Pathol 37:862-866.
Pothier L, Lane WW, et al., (1987). Plasma
  selenium levels in patients with advanced upper
  gastrointestinal cancer. Cancer 60:2251-2260.
Putzki H, Mlasowsky B, Duben W, (1985). Serum
  copper concentration no help in diagnosis of
  colorectal cancer? Clin Chem 31:352-352.
Rabinowitz MB, Levin SR, Gonick HC, (1980).
  Comparisons of chromium status in diabetic and
  normal men. Metabolism 4:355-364.
Robinson M, Godfrey PJ, et al., (1979). Blood
  selenium and glutathione, peroxidase activity in
  normal subjects and surgical patients with and
  without cancer in New Zealand. Am J Clin Nutr
  32:1477-1485.
Roguljic A, Roth A, Kolaric K, et al., (1980).
  Iron, copper and zinc liver tissue levels in
  patients with malignant lymphomas. Cancer
  46:565-569.
Shah-Reddy I, Khilanani P, Bishop CR, (1980).
  Serum copper levels in non-Hodgkin's lymphoma's.
  Cancer 45:2156-2159.
Sham I, Lewkow LM, Khilanani U, (1983).
  Correlation of hypercupremia with other acute
  phase reactants in malignant lymphoma. Cancer
  51:851-854.
Shamberger RJ, Rukovena E, Longfield AK, et al.,
  (1973). Antioxidants and cancer: I selenium in
  the blood of normals and cancer patients. J of
  the National Cancer Institute 50:863-870.
Shike M, Raulet M, et al., (1981). Copper
  metabolism and requirements in total parenteral
  nutrition. Gastroenterology 81:290-297.
Shroeder HA, (1967). Cadmium, chromium and
  cardiovascular disease. Circulation 35:570-582.
Solomons NW, (1985). Biochemical, metabolic and
  clinical role of copper in human nutrition.
  J Am Coll Nutr 4:83-105.

Sullivan JF, Heary RP, (1970). Zinc metabolism in alcoholic liver disease. Am J Clin Nutr 23:170-177.

Tengrup I, Samuelsson H, (1977). Changes in serum zinc during and after surgical procedures. Acta Chir Scand 143:195-99.

Tsukamoto Y, Iwanami S, and Marumo F, (1980). Nephron, disturbances of trace element concentrations in plasma in patients with chronic renal failure 26:174-179.

Tulikoura I, Vuori E, (1986). Effect of total parenteral nutrition on the zinc, copper and manganese status of patients with catabolic disease. Scand J Gastroenterol 21:421-27.

Valberg LS, Flanagan PR, Ghent CN, et al., (1985). Zinc absorption and leukocyte zinc in alcoholic and nonalcoholic cirrhosis. Dig Dis Sci 30:329-333.

Versieck J, Barbier I, Speecke A, et al., (1974). Manganese, copper, and zinc concentrations in serum and packed blood cells during acute hepatitis, chronic hepatitis, and posthepatic cirrhosis. Clin Chem 20:1141-1145.

Wabilach S, (1985). Clinical and biochemical aspects of chromium deficiency. J Am Coll Nutr 4:107-120.

Mineral Homeostasis in the Elderly, pages 245–250
© 1989 Alan R. Liss, Inc.

A MODEL FOR EFFECTIVE THERAPY FOR OSTEOPOROSIS

Marc K. Drezner, M.D.

Department of Medicine, Duke University
Medical Center, Durham, North
Carolina 27710

Effective therapy for osteoporosis depends on maintaining or establishing bone mass at a level sufficient to prevent fracture. Success in this regard has been largely limited to therapeutic agents (such as oral calcium, estrogen, calcitonin and diphosphonates) which inhibit bone resorption and thereby slow loss of bone mass. These agents have the prophylactic value of maintaining bone density, rather than the restorative value of replacing previously lost calcified tissue volume. Although these drugs have been successful, use of these agents has been limited by the inability to select the appropriate time at which physicians should initiate therapy in subjects of an as yet undefined population at risk for osteoporosis. In addition, contraindications in individual patients to the various forms of available treatment often decrease use of these drugs. Therefore, presentation of patients with decreased bone mass and established osteoporosis remains a common medical problem.

Unfortunately, returning bone mass to normal after osteoporosis has developed remains, in general, an elusive therapeutic goal. While sodium flouride therapy exhibits some value in increasing the calcified tissue volume in affected patients, the response is highly variable and unpredictable. The cause of such inconsistency remains ill-defined. However, since the sodium fluoride exerts its effects by stimulating bone formation at existing mineralized surfaces, a significant reduction in bone surface density may limit responsiveness.

If this were the case, effective treatment of osteoporosis would depend upon discovery of a therapeutic agent which stimulates bone formation along quiescent bone surfaces, as well as at independent sites within the marrow space. Such an effect would result in a significant increase of both trabecular bone volume and trabecular number which would correct the diminished bone mass characteristic of osteoporosis. Until recently, many experts believed that pharmacologic induction of such a formative process, de novo bone histogenesis, could not be achieved (Parfitt et al.). Rather, they felt that bone formation of this type remained solely a physiologic process which underlies primitive bone formation and fracture healing in man.

However, current studies in my laboratory (Quarles et al., 1987) indicate that uncoupled bone formation may be stimulated by mitogenic agents. In our investigations we assessed the effects of aluminum on bone remodeling in adult dogs to whom we administered aluminum chloride intravenously three times per week at doses of 0.75 mg/kg or 1.20 mg/kg. Bone histomorphology and serum biochemistries in these treated animals were compared with those in age-matched normals. Administration of aluminum at the relatively low dose resulted in a significant elevation of the serum aluminum concentration in treated beagles (151.7 ± 19.9 ug/l) compared to that in controls (4.2 ± 1.35 ug/l). In contrast, therapy did not significantly alter the serum total and ionized calcium, creatinine, iPTH, calcitriol or alkaline phosphatase levels after 8 or 16 weeks of treatment. Nevertheless, the serum phosphorus concentrations declined significantly at each interval.

Of more importance, in response to this regimen unique alterations developed in the bone of treated animals after 16 weeks. Biopsies from these dogs displayed evidence of de novo bone formation marked by buds of new lamellar bone at previously inactive surfaces and arborization of trabeculae. Consistent with these observations, a significant increase in bone volume and trabecular number was manifest compared to that in controls. In concert with these changes early evidence of peritrabecular fibrosis became apparent. These histologic changes were associated with an increment of bone aluminum and bone surface aluminum above that maintained in normal animals.

In contrast, administration of the higher dose of aluminum increased the serum aluminum concentration (1242.3$\pm$259.8 ug/1) to a level significantly greater than that in controls, as well as the dogs treated with a lower dose. However, high-dose treatment for 8 and 16 weeks, similar to a low-dose regimen, did not result in an alteration of serum total and ionized calcium, alkaline phosphatase, iPTH or calcitriol, but did decrease the serum phosphorus.

More significantly, after 8 weeks of treatment with this high-dose regimen, bone biopsies from the animals displayed changes similar to, but in many respects more pronounced than, those evidenced after 16 weeks of low-dose therapy. In this regard, a more abundant arborization of trabecular bone and consequent increased trabecular plate density and bone volume again provided evidence of enhanced de novo bone formation. In contrast, in this instance poorly mineralized woven bone (osteoid) constituted the majority of the newly synthesized tissue, comprising 11.5$\pm$4.6% of the bone volume. The presence of woven bone and a coincident increase in the number of osteoblasts within the tissue indicated that an accelerated rate of matrix synthesis had provided the impetus for new bone formation. Indeed, the concomitant appearance of marrow fibrosis provided further evidence that aluminum-induced mesenchymal cell proliferation (and differentiation) was responsible for the observed changes. These complex alterations occurred in association with a concomitant reduction in active bone resorption and an increase of the bone aluminum content and aluminum-covered bone surfaces.

Continuation of high-dose aluminum treatment for up to 16 weeks resulted in further de novo bone formation. Bone volume continued to increase as did the trabecular number. In addition, mineralization of bone was more complete, largely reflecting calcification of woven bone. These changes occurred in spite of further aluminum accumulation on bone surfaces and sustenance of bone aluminum content.

The data from this study clearly illustrate that aluminum administration stimulates uncoupled bone formation and induces a positive bone balance in adult beagles which exhibit bone remodeling dynamics similar to that in man. Although many questions remain about the mechanisms of action, potential marrow toxicity (secondary to peritrabecular fibrosis), bone strength, remodeling of woven bone, and the ability to sustain the increased volume, aluminum appears to be a pharmacologic (mitogenic) agent which can increase osteoblast number, stimulate osteoblastic collagen synthesis, and thereby induce de novo bone histogenesis. As such, aluminum may serve as a model for the development of a potentially effective therapy for osteoporosis which has, to date, remained elusive.

More recently, we have begun to further develop this model. In this regard, we have examined the influence of osteoblast function on the aluminum induced de novo bone histogenesis (Quarles et al., 1988). We chose to alter this variable because bone from patients with osteoporosis generally exhibits a diminished pool of active osteoblasts. Thus, stimulation of uncoupled bone formation may be limited in this disease if pharmacologic induction of a bone trophic response is dependent upon this cell population. Since studies of parathyroid hormone effects on replication of pre-osteoblasts in dogs in vivo (Malluche et al., 1988) and proliferation of immature osteoblasts in vitro (Wong et al.) indicate that this hormone sustains the activity/number of the osteoblast pool, we designed our investigation to examine whether diminished osteoblast function secondary to parathyroid hormone deficiency limits aluminum action. Thyroparathyroidectomized dogs maintained normal plasma calcium and calcitriol levels secondary to dietary supplements but developed evidence of decreased osteoblast activity, including diminished osteoid covered trabecular bone surface and a decreased osteoblast number. Administration of aluminum (1.25 mg/kg) increased the serum aluminum levels in both sham and TPTX animals above normal but did not alter the calcium, creatinine or parathyoid hormone from control levels in either group. After 8 weeks of therapy, however, bone biopsies from sham-operated beagles displayed evidence of de novo bone histogenesis including an increased bone volume ($47.0\pm.0$ vs 30.4 ± 0.9) and trabecular number (4.1 ± 0.2 vs 3.2 ± 0.2 /mm). As before, much of the enhanced volume resulted from deposition of poorly mineralized woven bone ($9.9\pm2.7\%$). In contrast, biopsies from aluminum treated TPTX animals exhibited significantly less evidence of ectopic bone formation. In this regard, bone ($35.5\pm1.7\%$) and woven tissue volume ($1.4\pm0.8\%$), as well as trabecular number (3.3 ± 0.1/mm) were significantly less than those of the aluminum treated controls. These observations indicate that osteoblast quiescence attenuates aluminum induced de novo bone histogenesis. Therefore, successful application of such a stimulus to evoke bone formation in patients with osteoporosis may depend upon pre-treatment designed to increase the functional osteoblast pool.

In any case, our observations provide the initial basis for developing an effective treatment for osteoporosis. Demonstration that drug induced de novo bone histogenesis can be achieved indicates that refurbishment of bone volume in patients with osteopenia is a potential reality. While such a success may depend upon increasing osteoblast activity a priori, it should not be limited by a diminished bone surface/volume ratio. Consequently, the failure associated with fluoride therapy may be circumvented. Nevertheless, we recognize that aluminum per se is unlikely the drug which will or should be used as a treatment modality for osteoporosis. A variety of potential toxicities, as well as dependence upon an intravenous route of administration, mitigate against employing this agent as a therapy of choice. Rather, we feel that treatment modalities may be developed that either mimic aluminum effects by an independent mechanism or activate the pathway of aluminum action at a point distal to those events which result in negative effects. Regardless, de novo bone histogenesis may well be the mechanism which underlies the first truely effective treatment for established osteoporosis.

REFERENCES

Malluche HH, Sherman D, Meyer W, Ritz E, Norman AW, Massry SG (1982). Effects of long-term infusion of physiologic doses of 1-34 PTH on bone. Am. J. Physiol. 242:F1979-F2001.

Parfitt AM, Matthews CHE, Villanueva AR, Kleerekoper M, Frame B, Rao DS (1983). Relationship between surface, volume and thickness of iliac trabecular bone in aging and osteoporosis: Implications for the microanatomic and cellular mechanism of bone loss. J. Clin. Invest. 72:1396-1409.

Quarles LD, Gitelman HJ, Drezner MK (1987). Aluminum induced de novo bone formation: Modulation by parathyroid hormone. J. Bone Min. Res 2:(Suppl 1)401 (Abstract).

Quarles LD, Gitelman HJ, Drezner MK (1988). Induction of de novo bone formation in the beagle: A novel effect of aluminum. J. Clin. Invest. 81:1056–1066.

Wong GL (1986). Skeletal effects of parathyroid hormonel. In: Bone and Mineral Research W.A. Peck, editor. Elsevier Science Publishing Co., Inc., New York., 103–129.

Mineral Homeostasis in the Elderly, pages 251–255
© 1989 Alan R. Liss, Inc.

Research Summary:

OSTEOPOROSIS: A MULTIDISCIPLINARY PROGRAM OF PREVENTION AND
THERAPY

Connie W. Bales, Deborah T. Gold, Kenneth W. Lyles
and Marc K. Drezner, Center for the Study of Aging
and Human Development and Departments of Medicine,
Physiology, and Psychiatry, Duke University
Medical Center, and GRECC, Veterans Administration
Hospital, Durham, NC   27710

INTRODUCTION

Osteoporosis, a chronic metabolic bone disease characterized by non-traumatic fractures, debilitation and pain,
has moved to the forefront of public awareness. Concern has
been expressed not only for the 25-35 million Americans
already affected by osteoporosis, but also for the antici-
pated increase in incidence of this disease as the number
and proportion of older adults in the population grows to a
record high in the twenty-first century (Melton and Riggs,
1987).

In response to increasing recognition of the prevalence
and severity of osteoporosis, programs designed to prevent
and/or treat this disease have been developed at a number of
medical centers across the United States. These programs can
implement recent improvements in the approach to osteoporosis
management and treatment (Bone HG, 1986). However, it is now
clear that osteoporosis is a complex disorder of multiple
types with different etiologies (Kleerekoper M, 1986). For
this reason, therapeutic programs aimed at prevention of bone
loss and/or improvement of existing conditions must be
tailored to the characteristics of the individual patient.
Modification of the treatment program according to the age
and sex of the patient, co-morbidity and associated therapies, and availability of family and other social support
thus becomes an essential component of effective long-term
management. Because patients differ in response to, and
tolerance for, various types of therapy, the efficacy of the
prescribed treatment must be monitored on a long-term basis
and therapeutic strategies continually modified as necessary.

This paper outlines a program of therapy for osteoporosis, the Duke Preventive and Therapeutic Program for Osteoporosis (DUPATPO), which has been established recently at Duke University Medical Center for patients with osteoporosis and those judged to be at high risk for the disease. This program is unique in its multidisciplinary approach to osteoporosis management, attending to both the physical and emotional needs of the patient through a highly individualized therapeutic plan. In addition, continuity of care is provided by scheduling follow-up evaluations at regular intervals for a minimum of two years post-program.

PROGRAM DESCRIPTION

Patients screened from referrals to the Bone and Mineral Metabolism Clinic at Duke Medical Center may elect to participate in an intensive four-day regimen (DUPATPO) which consolidates appropriate diagnostic procedures, physical therapy, nutritional and medical intervention, and training for lifestyle modification into a cohesive and individualized program of therapy. The primary goal of this prevention/treatment program is to ameliorate both physiological and psychological stresses caused by osteoporosis (Figure 1).

Specialty areas represented by the program staff include endocrinology, geriatrics, physical therapy, nutrition, and medical sociology. Consultants from orthopedics, rheumatology, cardiology, nuclear medicine, and radiology compliment the core staff. Initial diagnostic procedures for all new patients include routine blood and urine chemistries, as well as measurements of hormone/metabolic factors which may influence bone remodeling. Radiologic studies include densitometric evaluation of trabecular/cortical bone and other radiographs as indicated.

Physical therapy evaluation and treadmill testing precede a minimum of six hours of individualized instruction in appropriate exercise and activity programs. In addition, dietary evaluation based upon a 3-day diet record and food frequency questionnaire provides the basis for the implementation of a nutritional care plan developed by a registered dietitian. Instructional sessions presented by the professional staff during the program help patients to learn the facts about osteoporosis and lifestyle changes which can prevent further progression of the disease. Patients are taught to modify their diets, to initiate a regular program of physical exercise, to safely perform activities of daily living and to take advantage of devices such as braces, reachers, and safety handholds to minimize the risk of falls and undue skeletal stress. In addition, patients are encouraged to utilize social supports such as family and friends and pursue an active lifestyle. These suggestions help patients to normalize their condition as much as possible and to engage in appropriate coping processes (Lazarus and Folkman, 1984). The individualized care provided during these sessions is an essential component of the DUPATPO approach to managing chronic disability. Routine follow-ups at 3, 12 and 24 months provide contact with the professional staff and allow for reinforcement of prescribed therapies and emotional support.

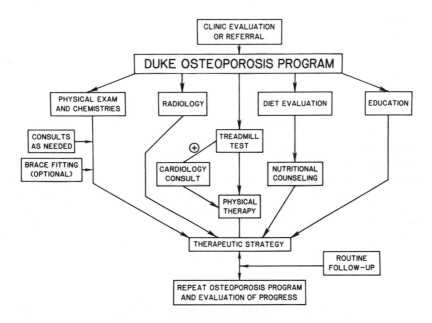

Figure 1. Schematic diagram of multidisciplinary approach to osteoporosis management. All steps are routine, with the exception of brace fitting (which is a function of patient need and preference) and the cardiology consult (which is initiated only if the result of the treadmill test is positive).

SUMMARY OF PROGRAM OUTCOMES

Due to increasing awareness of the prevalence of
osteoporosis by health care professionals and the lay community, interest in DUPATPO has grown continuously since the
program's inception. Current patient census suggests that
enrollment will at least double within this calendar year.

To date, the relatively small number of patients who
have completed more than one year of therapy limits our ability to conduct valid statistical evaluations of medical
progress. However, it is clear from informal observations
at intermediate follow-ups that an obvious improvement in
physical condition (including appropriate changes in body
weight and amount of pain medication routinely required)
occurs in many patients during the first 3 to 6 months
post-program. In fact, in many instances, physical progress and improvement in morale are noted within the time
frame of the initial 4-day program. Other indicators of
program effectiveness include improvement in dietary calcium intake and enhanced general and spinal mobility, a
change attributed to the effects of the intensive program
of physical therapy developed for each patient.

Although DUPATPO does not directly address the psychoso-
cial stress of chronic disease, it has become obvious to clinic staff that patients have improved psychological as well
as physical outcomes after program participation. Analyses
of data collected during the four-day program indicate a
marked improvement in understanding of the disease and more
frequent use of appropriate coping strategies. Patients
demonstrate a definite improvement ($p<0.0001$) in factual
knowledge concerning osteoporosis (as measured by pre- and
post-tests) and report substantial reductions in feelings of
depression between the initiation and completion of the
program (Gold et al., 1988).

In summary, the effectiveness of our program of therapy
for osteoporosis is clearly linked to its focus on treating
the needs of the "whole" patient. Physicians have long recognized that a positive attitude and optimistic compliance
with therapeutic recommendations contribute to the successful management of chronic disease. Based upon our experience
thus far, we strongly recommend that the treatment of
osteoporosis be founded upon a multidisciplinary approach
which helps patients optimize quality of life by meeting both
physical and emotional needs.

REFERENCES

Bone HG (1986). The future of osteoporosis therapy. In Posen
    S (ed): "A Discussion of the Diagnosis and Treatment of
    Osteoporosis," Toronto: Hans Huber Publishers, pp 64-66.

Gold DT, Bales CW, Lyles KW, Drezner MK. Unexpected
    outcomes: The psychological impact of a medical educa-
    tion program on osteoporosis patients. Under review.

Kleerekoper M (1986). Are there difference types of
    osteoporosis and does it matter? In Posen S (ed): "A
    Discussion of the Diagnosis and Treatment of
    Osteoporosis," Toronto: Hans Huber Publishers, pp 51-55.

Lazarus RS, Folkman S (1984). Coping and adaptation. In
    Gentry WD (ed): "The Handbook of Behavioral Medicine,"
    New York: Guilford Press, pp 282-325.

Melton LJ, Riggs BL (1987). Epidemiology of age-related
    fractures. In Avioli LV (ed): "The Osteoporosis
    Syndrome: Detection, Prevention, and Treatment," 2nd ed.,
    Orlando: Grune & Stratton, Inc., pp 1-30.

Index

and cell differentiation, 75
cellular levels in elderly subjects, 87
competition with cations, 82
and copper absorption, 56–57, 182
deficiency of, 47, 69, 177–182
   in acrodermatitis enteropathica, 71–72, 79, 213
   biochemical effects of, 201–204
   clinical features of, 72–74
   dark adaptation in, 72
   dermatological signs of, 73
   drug-induced, 71
   in elderly subjects, 82–83
   etiology of, 70–72
   in liver disease, 71, 226–227
   in malabsorption syndrome, 71, 73
   neuropsychiatric disorders in, 73
   in parenteral nutrition, 72
   in pregnancy, 74
   in sickle cell disease, 71, 72, 79–80
   testosterone levels in, 76–77, 87–88
dietary intakes of, 149–151, 171–173
   recommended, 4–5, 151–153
and DNA synthesis, 75

and free-radical reactions, 81–82, 216
and gene expression, 76
and gonadal function, 76–77
in host defense processes, 213–216
in immune function, 40, 78–82, 84–89, 179–180, 213–215
interaction with calcium, 77–78, 82
interaction with copper, 92, 146–147, 148
leukocyte levels of, 177
and lipid peroxidation, 216
and platelet aggregation, 77
redistribution in tissues, 215
   in disease states, 226
requirements of elderly subjects
   disease affecting, 173–174
   medications affecting, 174
and RNA synthesis, 75
role in nutrition, 40
serum levels of, 150, 175, 176
   in disease states, 226–230
and taste acuity, 73, 83, 178
therapeutic uses of, 150, 175–177
tolerance test, 50–52
and wound healing, 73, 83–84, 178–179

DATE DUE

FEB 10 1994			
JAN 11 1995			
APR 17 1995			
APR 10 1996			